The Gift of
Therapy

The Gift of
Therapy

AN OPEN LETTER TO A NEW GENERATION

OF THERAPISTS AND THEIR PATIENTS

Irvin D. Yalom, M.D.

*HarperCollins*Publishers

HarperCollins books may be purchased for educational, business, or sales promotional use. For information, please write: Special Markets Department, HarperCollins Publishers Inc., 10 East 53rd Street, New York, NY 10022.

Printed on acid-free paper

FIRST EDITION

Designed by Nicola Ferguson

Library of Congress Cataloging-in-Publication Data
Yalom, Irvin D.
The gift of therapy : an open letter to a new generation
of therapists and their patients / Irvin D. Yalom.
p.   cm.
Includes bibliographical references and index.
ISBN 0-06-621440-8
1. Psychotherapy.   2. Psychotherapist and patient.
3. Yalom, Irvin D.   I. Title.
RC480 .Y35   2002
616.89'14—dc21   2001039319

02   03   04   05   06   10   9   8   7   6   5   4   3   2   1

to Marilyn,
soul mate for over fifty years.
still counting.

CONTENTS

Introduction

It is dark. I come to your office but can't find you. Your office is empty. I enter and look around. The only thing there is your Panama hat. And it is all filled with cobwebs.

My patients' dreams have changed. Cobwebs fill my hat. My office is dark and deserted. I am nowhere to be found.

My patients worry about my health: Will I be there for the long haul of therapy? When I leave for vacation, they fear I will never return. They imagine attending my funeral or visiting my grave.

My patients do not let me forget that I grow old. But they are only doing their job: Have I not asked them to disclose all feelings, thoughts, and dreams? Even potential new patients join the chorus and, without fail, greet me with the question: "Are you *still* taking on patients?"

One of our chief modes of death denial is a belief in personal *specialness*, a conviction that we are exempt from biological necessity and that life will not deal with us in the same harsh way it deals with everyone else. I remember, many years ago, visiting an optometrist because of diminishing vision. He asked my age and then responded: "Forty-eight, eh? Yep, you're right on schedule!"

Of course I knew, consciously, that he was entirely correct, but a cry welled up from deep within: "What schedule? *Who's* on schedule? It is altogether right that you and others may be on schedule, but certainly not I!"

And so it is daunting to realize that I am entering a designated later era of life. My goals, interests, and ambitions are changing in predictable fashion. Erik Erikson, in his study of the life cycle, described this late-life stage as *generativity*, a post-narcissism era when attention turns from expansion of oneself toward care and concern for succeeding generations. Now, as I have reached seventy, I can appreciate the clarity of Erikson's vision. His concept of generativity feels right to me. I want to pass on what I have learned. And as soon as possible.

But offering guidance and inspiration to the next generation of psychotherapists is exceedingly problematic today, because our field is in such crisis. An economically driven health-care system mandates a radical modification in psychological treatment, and psychotherapy is now obliged to be streamlined—that is, above all, *inexpensive* and, perforce, brief, superficial, and insubstantial.

I worry where the next generation of effective psychotherapists will be trained. Not in psychiatry residency training programs. Psychiatry is on the verge of abandoning the field of psychotherapy. Young psychiatrists are forced to specialize in psychopharmacology because third-party payers now reimburse for psychotherapy only if it is delivered by low-fee (in other words, minimally trained) practitioners. It seems certain that the present generation of psychiatric clinicians, skilled in both dynamic psychotherapy and in pharmacological treatment, is an endangered species.

What about clinical psychology training programs—the obvious choice to fill the gap? Unfortunately, clinical psychologists face the same market pressures, and most doctorate-granting schools of psychology are responding by teaching a therapy that is symptom-oriented, brief, and, hence, reimbursable.

So I worry about psychotherapy—about how it may be deformed by economic pressures and impoverished by radically abbreviated training programs. Nonetheless, I am confident that, in the future, a cohort of therapists coming from a variety of educational disciplines (psychology, counseling, social work, pastoral counseling, clinical philosophy) will continue to pursue rigorous postgraduate training and, even in the crush of HMO reality, will find patients desiring extensive growth and change willing to make an open-ended commitment to therapy. It is for these therapists and these patients that I write *The Gift of Therapy*.

THROUGHOUT THESE PAGES I advise students against sectarianism and suggest a therapeutic pluralism in which effective interventions are drawn from several different therapy approaches. Still, for the most part, I work from an interpersonal and existential frame of reference. Hence, the bulk of the advice that follows issues from one or the other of these two perspectives.

Since first entering the field of psychiatry, I have had two abiding interests: group therapy and existential therapy. These are parallel but separate interests: I do not practice "existential group therapy"—in fact, I don't know what that would be. The two modes are different not only because of the format (that is, a group of approximately six to nine members versus a one-to-one setting for existential psychotherapy) but in their fundamental *frame of reference*. When I see patients in group therapy I work from an interpersonal frame of reference and make the assumption that patients fall into despair because of their inability to develop and sustain gratifying interpersonal relationships.

However, when I operate from an existential frame of reference, I make a very different assumption: patients fall into despair as a result of a confrontation with harsh facts of the human condition—the "givens" of existence. Since many of the offerings in this book issue from an existential framework that is unfamiliar to many readers, a brief introduction is in order.

Definition of existential psychotherapy: *Existential psychotherapy is a dynamic therapeutic approach that focuses on concerns rooted in existence.*

Let me dilate this terse definition by clarifying the phrase "dynamic approach." *Dynamic* has both a lay and technical definition. The lay meaning of *dynamic* (derived from the Greek root *dynasthai,* to have power or strength) implying forcefulness or vitality (to wit, *dynamo,* a dynamic football runner or political orator) is obviously not relevant here. But if that were the meaning, applied to our profession, then where is the therapist who would claim to be other than a dynamic therapist, in other words, a sluggish or inert therapist?

No, I use "dynamic" in its *technical* sense, which retains the idea of force but is rooted in Freud's model of mental functioning, positing that *forces* in conflict within the individual generate the individual's thought, emotion, and behavior. Furthermore—and this is a crucial point—*these conflicting forces exist at varying levels of awareness; indeed some are entirely unconscious.*

So existential psychotherapy is a dynamic therapy that, like the various psychoanalytic therapies, assumes that unconscious forces influence conscious functioning. However, it parts company from the various psychoanalytic ideologies when we ask the next question: What is the nature of the conflicting internal forces?

The existential psychotherapy approach posits that the inner conflict bedeviling us issues not only from our struggle with suppressed instinctual strivings or internalized significant adults or shards of forgotten traumatic memories, but also *from our confrontation with the "givens" of existence.*

And what are these "givens" of existence? If we permit ourselves to screen out or "bracket" the everyday concerns of life and reflect deeply upon our situation in the world, we inevitably arrive at the deep structures of existence (the "ultimate concerns," to use theologian Paul Tillich's term). Four ultimate concerns, to my view, are highly salient to psychotherapy: death, isolation, meaning in life, and freedom. (Each of these ultimate concerns will be defined and discussed in a designated section.)

Students have often asked why I don't advocate training programs in existential psychotherapy. The reason is that *I've never considered existential psychotherapy to be a discrete, freestanding ideological school.* Rather than attempt to develop existential psychotherapy curricula, I prefer to supplement the education of all well-trained dynamic therapists by increasing their *sensibility to existential issues.*

Process and content. What does existential therapy look like in practice? To answer that question one must attend to both "content" and "process," the two major aspects of therapy discourse. "Content" is just what it says—the precise words spoken, the substantive issues addressed. "Process" refers to an entirely different and enormously important dimension: the interpersonal relationship between the patient and therapist.

When we ask about the "process" of an interaction, we mean: What do the words (and the nonverbal behavior as well) tell us about the nature of the relationship between the parties engaged in the interaction?

If my therapy sessions were observed, one might often look in vain for lengthy explicit discussions of death, freedom, meaning, or existential isolation. Such existential *content* may be salient for only some (but not all) patients at some (but not all) stages of therapy. In fact, the effective therapist should never try to force discussion of any content area: *Therapy should not be theory-driven but relationship-driven.*

But observe these same sessions for some characteristic *process* deriving from an existential orientation and one will encounter another story entirely. A heightened sensibility to existential issues deeply *influences the nature of the relationship of the therapist and patient and affects every single therapy session.*

I myself am surprised by the particular form this book has taken. I never expected to author a book containing a sequence of tips for therapists. Yet, looking back, I know the precise moment of inception. Two years ago, after viewing the Huntington Japanese gardens in Pasadena, I noted the Huntington Library's exhibit of best-selling books from the Renaissance in Great Britain and wandered in. Three of the ten exhibited volumes were books of numbered "tips"—on animal husbandry, sewing, gardening. I was struck that even then, hundreds of years ago, just after the introduction of the printing press, lists of tips attracted the attention of the multitudes.

Years ago, I treated a writer who, having flagged in the writing of two consecutive novels, resolved never to undertake another book until one came along and bit her on the ass. I chuckled at her remark but didn't really comprehend what she meant until that moment in the Huntington Library when the idea of a book of tips bit me on the ass. On the spot, I resolved to put away other writing projects, to begin looting my clinical notes and journals, and to write an open letter to beginning therapists.

Rainer Maria Rilke's ghost hovered over the writing of this volume. Shortly before my experience in the Huntington Library, I had reread his *Letters to a Young Poet* and I have consciously attempted to raise myself to his standards of honesty, inclusiveness, and generosity of spirit.

The advice in this book is drawn from notes of forty-five years of clinical practice. It is an idiosyncratic mélange of ideas and techniques that I have found useful in my work. These ideas are so personal, opinionated, and occasionally original that the reader is unlikely to encounter them elsewhere. Hence, this volume is in no way meant to be a systematic manual; I intend it instead as a supplement to a comprehensive training program. I selected the eighty-five categories in this volume randomly, guided by my passion for the task rather than by any particular order or system. I began with a list of more than two hundred pieces of advice, and ultimately pruned away those for which I felt too little enthusiasm.

One other factor influenced my selection of these eighty-five items. My recent novels and stories contain many descriptions of therapy procedures I've found useful in my clinical work but, since my fiction has a comic, often burlesque tone, it is unclear to many readers whether I am serious about the therapy procedures I describe. *The Gift of Therapy* offers me an opportunity to set the record straight.

As a nuts-and-bolts collection of favorite interventions or statements, this volume is long on technique and short on theory. Readers seeking more theoretical background may wish to read my texts *Existential Psychotherapy* and *The Theory and Practice of Group Psychotherapy,* the mother books for this work.

Being trained in medicine and psychiatry, I have grown

accustomed to the term *patient* (from the Latin *patiens*—one who suffers or endures) but I use it synonymously with *client,* the common appellation of psychology and counseling traditions. To some, the term *patient* suggests an aloof, disinterested, unengaged, authoritarian therapist stance. But read on—I intend to encourage throughout a therapeutic relationship based on engagement, openness, and egalitarianism.

Many books, my own included, consist of a limited number of substantive points and then considerable filler to connect the points in a graceful manner. Because I have selected a large number of suggestions, many freestanding, and omitted much filler and transitions, the text will have an episodic, lurching quality.

Though I selected these suggestions haphazardly and expect many readers to sample these offerings in an unsystematic manner, I have tried, as an afterthought, to group them in a reader-friendly fashion.

The first section (1–40) addresses the nature of the therapist-patient relationship, with particular emphasis on the here-and-now, the therapist's use of the self, and therapist self-disclosure.

The next section (41–51) turns from process to *content* and suggests methods of exploring the ultimate concerns of death, meaning in life, and freedom (encompassing responsibility and decision).

The third section (52–76) addresses a variety of issues arising in the everyday conduct of therapy.

In the fourth section (77–83) I address the use of dreams in therapy.

The final section (84–85) discusses the hazards and privileges of being a therapist.

This text is sprinkled with many of my favorite specific

phrases and interventions. At the same time I encourage spontaneity and creativity. *Hence do not view my idiosyncratic interventions as a specific procedural recipe; they represent my own
perspective and my attempt to reach inside to find my own style
and voice.* Many students will find that other theoretical positions and technical styles will prove more compatible for them.
The advice in this book derives from my clinical practice with
moderately high- to high-functioning patients (rather than
those who are psychotic or markedly disabled) meeting once or,
less commonly, twice a week, for a few months to two to three
years. My therapy goals with these patients are ambitious: in
addition to symptom removal and alleviation of pain, I strive to
facilitate personal growth and basic character change. I know
that many of my readers may have a different clinical situation:
a different setting with a different patient population and a
briefer duration of therapy. Still it is my hope that readers find
their own creative way to adapt and apply what I have learned
to their own particular work situation.

Acknowledgments

Many have assisted me in the writing of this book. First, as always, I am much indebted to my wife, Marilyn, always my first and most thorough reader. Several colleagues read and expertly critiqued the entire manuscript: Murray Bilmes, Peter Rosenbaum, David Spiegel, Ruthellen Josselson, and Saul Spiro. A number of colleagues and students critiqued parts of the manuscript: Neil Brast, Rick Van Rheenen, Martel Bryant, Ivan Gendzel, Randy Weingarten, Ines Roe, Evelyn Beck, Susan Goldberg, Tracy Larue Yalom, and Scott Haigley. Members of my professional support group generously granted me considerable air time to discuss sections of this book. Several of my patients permitted me to include incidents and dreams from their therapy. To all, my gratitude.

CHAPTER I

Remove the Obstacles to Growth

When I was finding my way as a young psychotherapy student, the most useful book I read was Karen Horney's *Neurosis and Human Growth*. And the single most useful concept in that book was the notion that the human being has an inbuilt propensity toward self-realization. If obstacles are removed, Horney believed, the individual will develop into a mature, fully realized adult, just as an acorn will develop into an oak tree.

"Just as an acorn develops into an oak . . ." What a wonderfully liberating and clarifying image! It forever changed my approach to psychotherapy by offering me a new vision of my work: My task was to remove obstacles blocking my patient's path. I did not have to do the entire job; I did not have to inspirit the patient with the desire to grow, with curiosity, will, zest for life, caring, loyalty, or any of the myriad of characteristics that make us fully human. No, what I had to do was to identify and remove obstacles. The rest would follow automatically, fueled by the self-actualizing forces within the patient.

I remember a young widow with, as she put it, a "failed heart"—an inability ever to love again. It felt daunting to address the inability to love. I didn't know how to do that. But dedicating myself to identifying and uprooting her many blocks to loving? I could do that.

I soon learned that love felt treasonous to her. To love another was to betray her dead husband; it felt to her like pounding the final nails in her husband's coffin. To love another as deeply as she did her husband (and she would settle for nothing less) meant that her love for her husband had been in some way insufficient or flawed. To love another would be self-destructive because loss, and the searing pain of loss, was inevitable. To love again felt irresponsible: she was evil and jinxed, and her kiss was the kiss of death.

We worked hard for many months to identify all these obstacles to her loving another man. For months we wrestled with each irrational obstacle in turn. But once that was done, the patient's internal processes took over: she met a man, she fell in love, she married again. I didn't have to teach her to search, to give, to cherish, to love—I wouldn't have known how to do that.

A few words about Karen Horney: Her name is unfamiliar to most young therapists. Because the shelf life of eminent theorists in our field has grown so short, I shall, from time to time, lapse into reminiscence—not merely for the sake of paying homage but to emphasize the point that our field has a long history of remarkably able contributors who have laid deep foundations for our therapy work today.

One uniquely American addition to psychodynamic theory is embodied in the "neo-Freudian" movement—a group of clinicians and theorists who reacted against Freud's original focus on drive theory, that is, the notion that the developing individual is largely controlled by the unfolding and expression of inbuilt drives.

Instead, the neo-Freudians emphasized that we consider the vast influence of the interpersonal environment that envelops the individual and that, throughout life, shapes character structure. The best-known interpersonal theorists, Harry Stack Sullivan, Erich Fromm, and Karen Horney, have been so deeply integrated and assimilated into our therapy language and practice that we are all, without knowing it, neo-Freudians. One is reminded of Monsieur Jourdain in Molière's *Le Bourgeois Gentilhomme,* who, upon learning the definition of "prose," exclaims with wonderment, "To think that all my life I've been speaking prose without knowing it."

CHAPTER 2

Avoid Diagnosis
(*Except for Insurance Companies*)

Today's psychotherapy students are exposed to too much emphasis on diagnosis. Managed-care administrators demand that therapists arrive quickly at a precise diagnosis and then proceed upon a course of brief, focused therapy that matches that particular diagnosis. Sounds good. Sounds logical and efficient. But it has precious little to do with reality. It represents instead an illusory attempt to legislate scientific precision into being when it is neither possible nor desirable.

Though diagnosis is unquestionably critical in treatment considerations for many severe conditions with a biological substrate (for example, schizophrenia, bipolar disorders, major affective disorders, temporal lobe epilepsy, drug toxicity, organic or brain disease from toxins, degenerative causes, or infectious agents), diagnosis is often *counterproductive* in the everyday psychotherapy of less severely impaired patients.

Why? For one thing, psychotherapy consists of a gradual unfolding process wherein the therapist attempts to know the patient as fully as possible. A diagnosis limits vision; it diminishes ability to relate to the other as a person. Once we make a diagnosis, we tend to selectively inattend to aspects of the patient that do not fit into that particular diagnosis, and correspondingly overattend to subtle features that appear to confirm an initial diagnosis. What's more, a diagnosis may act as a self-fulfilling prophecy. Relating to a patient as a "borderline" or a "hysteric" may serve to stimulate and perpetuate those very traits. Indeed, there is a long history of iatrogenic influence on the shape of clinical entities, including the current controversy about multiple-personality disorder and repressed memories of sexual abuse. And keep in mind, too, the low reliability of the DSM personality disorder category (the very patients often engaging in longer-term psychotherapy).

And what therapist has not been struck by how much easier it is to make a DSM-IV diagnosis following the first interview than much later, let us say, after the tenth session, when we know a great deal more about the individual? Is this not a strange kind of science? A colleague of mine brings this point home to his psychiatric residents by asking, "If you are in personal psychotherapy or are considering it, what DSM-IV diagnosis do you think your therapist could justifiably use to describe someone as complicated as you?"

In the therapeutic enterprise we must tread a fine line between some, but not too much, objectivity; if we take the DSM diagnostic system too seriously, if we really believe we are truly carving at the joints of nature, then we may threaten the human, the spontaneous, the creative and uncertain nature of the therapeutic venture. Remember that the clinicians involved in formulating previous, now discarded, diagnostic systems were competent, proud, and just as confident as the current members of the DSM committees. Undoubtedly the time will come when the DSM-IV Chinese restaurant menu format will appear ludicrous to mental health professionals.

CHAPTER 3

Therapist and Patient as "Fellow Travelers"

André Malraux, the French novelist, described a country priest who had taken confession for many decades and summed up what he had learned about human nature in this manner: "First of all, people are much more unhappy than one thinks . . . and there is no such thing as a grown-up person." Everyone—and that includes therapists as well as patients—is destined to experience not only the exhilaration of life, but also its inevitable darkness: disillusionment, aging, illness, isolation, loss, meaninglessness, painful choices, and death.

No one put things more starkly and more bleakly than the German philosopher Arthur Schopenhauer:

In early youth, as we contemplate our coming life, we are like children in a theater before the curtain is raised, sitting there in high spirits and eagerly waiting for the play to begin. It is a blessing that we do not know what is really going to happen. Could we foresee it, there are

times when children might seem like condemned prison-
ers, condemned, not to death, but to life, and as yet all
unconscious of what their sentence means.

Or again:

We are like lambs in the field, disporting themselves
under the eyes of the butcher, who picks out one first and
then another for his prey. So it is that in our good days we
are all unconscious of the evil that Fate may have
presently in store for us—sickness, poverty, mutilation,
loss of sight or reason.

Though Schopenhauer's view is colored heavily by his own
personal unhappiness, still it is difficult to deny the inbuilt
despair in the life of every self-conscious individual. My wife and
I have sometimes amused ourselves by planning imaginary din-
ner parties for groups of people sharing similar propensities—
for example, a party for monopolists, or flaming narcissists, or
artful passive-aggressives we have known or, conversely, a
"happy" party to which we invite only the truly happy people we
have encountered. Though we've encountered no problems fill-
ing all sorts of other whimsical tables, we've never been able to
populate a full table for our "happy people" party. Each time we
identify a few characterologically cheerful people and place
them on a waiting list while we continue our search to complete the table, we find that one or another of our happy guests
is eventually stricken by some major life adversity—often a
severe illness or that of a child or spouse.

This tragic but realistic view of life has long influenced my
relationship to those who seek my help. Though there are many
phrases for the therapeutic relationship (patient/therapist,
client/counselor, analysand/analyst, client/facilitator, and the

latest—and, by far, the most repulsive—user/provider), none of these phrases accurately convey my sense of the therapeutic relationship. Instead I prefer to think of my patients and myself as *fellow travelers,* a term that abolishes distinctions between "them" (the afflicted) and "us" (the healers). During my training I was often exposed to the idea of the fully analyzed therapist, but as I have progressed through life, formed intimate relationships with a good many of my therapist colleagues, met the senior figures in the field, been called upon to render help to my former therapists and teachers, and myself become a teacher and an elder, I have come to realize the mythic nature of this idea. We are all in this together and there is no therapist and no person immune to the inherent tragedies of existence.

One of my favorite tales of healing, found in Hermann Hesse's *Magister Ludi,* involves Joseph and Dion, two renowned healers, who lived in biblical times. Though both were highly effective, they worked in different ways. The younger healer, Joseph, healed through quiet, inspired listening. Pilgrims trusted Joseph. Suffering and anxiety poured into his ears vanished like water on the desert sand and penitents left his presence emptied and calmed. On the other hand, Dion, the older healer, actively confronted those who sought his help. He divined their unconfessed sins. He was a great judge, chastiser, scolder, and rectifier, and he healed through active intervention. Treating the penitents as children, he gave advice, punished by assigning penance, ordered pilgrimages and marriages, and compelled enemies to make up.

The two healers never met, and they worked as rivals for many years until Joseph grew spiritually ill, fell into dark despair, and was assailed with ideas of self-destruction. Unable to heal himself with his own therapeutic methods, he set out on a journey to the south to seek help from Dion.

On his pilgrimage, Joseph rested one evening at an oasis, where he fell into a conversation with an older traveler. When Joseph described the purpose and destination of his pilgrimage, the traveler offered himself as a guide to assist in the search for Dion. Later, in the midst of their long journey together the old traveler revealed his identity to Joseph. Mirabile dictu: he himself was Dion—the very man Joseph sought.

Without hesitation Dion invited his younger, despairing rival into his home, where they lived and worked together for many years. Dion first asked Joseph to be a servant. Later he elevated him to a student and, finally, to full colleagueship. Years later, Dion fell ill and on his deathbed called his young colleague to him in order to hear a confession. He spoke of Joseph's earlier terrible illness and his journey to old Dion to plead for help. He spoke of how Joseph had felt it was a miracle that his fellow traveler and guide turned out to be Dion himself.

Now that he was dying, the hour had come, Dion told Joseph, to break his silence about that miracle. Dion confessed that at the time it had seemed a miracle to him as well, for he, too, had fallen into despair. He, too, felt empty and spiritually dead and, unable to help himself, had set off on a journey to seek help. On the very night that they had met at the oasis he was on a pilgrimage to a famous healer named Joseph.

HESSE'S TALE HAS always moved me in a preternatural way. It strikes me as a deeply illuminating statement about giving and receiving help, about honesty and duplicity, and about the relationship between healer and patient. The two men received powerful help but in very different ways. The younger healer was nurtured, nursed, taught, mentored, and parented. The older healer, on the other hand, was helped through serving another, through obtaining a disciple from whom he received filial love, respect, and salve for his isolation.

But now, reconsidering the story, I question whether these two wounded healers could not have been of even more service to one another. Perhaps they missed the opportunity for something deeper, more authentic, more powerfully mutative. Perhaps the *real* therapy occurred at the deathbed scene, when they moved into honesty with the revelation that they were fellow travelers, both simply human, all too human. The twenty years of secrecy, helpful as they were, may have obstructed and prevented a more profound kind of help. What might have happened if Dion's deathbed confession had occurred twenty years earlier, if healer and seeker had joined together in facing the questions that have no answers?

All of this echoes Rilke's letters to a young poet in which he advises, "Have patience with everything unresolved and try to love the questions themselves." I would add: "Try to love the questioners as well."

CHAPTER 4

Engage the Patient

A great many of our patients have conflicts in the realm of intimacy, and obtain help in therapy sheerly through experiencing an intimate relationship with the therapist. Some fear intimacy because they believe there is something basically unacceptable about them, something repugnant and unforgivable. Given this, the act of revealing oneself fully to another and still being accepted may be the major vehicle of therapeutic help. Others may avoid intimacy because of fears of exploitation, colonization, or abandonment; for them, too, the intimate and caring therapeutic relationship that does not result in the anticipated catastrophe becomes a corrective emotional experience.

Hence, nothing takes precedence over the care and maintenance of my relationship to the patient, and I attend carefully to every nuance of how we regard each other. Does the patient seem distant today? Competitive? Inattentive to my comments? Does he make use of what I say in private but refuse to acknowledge my help openly? Is she overly respectful? Obse-

quious? Too rarely voicing any objection or disagreements?
Detached or suspicious? Do I enter his dreams or daydreams?
What are the words of imaginary conversations with me? All
these things I want to know, and more. I never let an hour go by
without checking into our relationship, sometimes with a simple statement like: "How are you and I doing today?" or "How
are you experiencing the space between us today?" Sometimes
I ask the patient to project herself into the future: "Imagine a
half hour from now—you're on your drive home, looking back
upon our session. How will you feel about you and me today?
What will be the unspoken statements or unasked questions
about our relationship today?"

CHAPTER 5

Be Supportive

One of the great values of obtaining intensive personal therapy is to experience for oneself the great value of positive support. Question: What do patients recall when they look back, years later, on their experience in therapy? Answer: Not insight, not the therapist's interpretations. More often than not, they remember the positive supportive statements of their therapist.

I make a point of regularly expressing my positive thoughts and feelings about my patients, along a wide range of attributes—for example, their social skills, intellectual curiosity, warmth, loyalty to their friends, articulateness, courage in facing their inner demons, dedication to change, willingness to self-disclose, loving gentleness with their children, commitment to breaking the cycle of abuse, and decision not to pass on the "hot potato" to the next generation. Don't be stingy—there's no point to it; there is every reason to express these observations and your positive sentiments. And beware of empty compliments—make your support as incisive as your feedback or interpretations. Keep in mind the therapist's great power—power that, in part, stems from our having been privy to our patients' most intimate life events, thoughts, and fantasies. Acceptance and support from one who knows you so intimately is enormously affirming.

If patients make an important and courageous therapeutic step, compliment them on it. If I've been deeply engaged in the hour and regret that it's come to an end, I say that I hate to bring this hour to an end. And (a confession—every therapist has a store of small secret transgressions!) I do not hesitate to express this nonverbally by running over the hour a few minutes.

Often the therapist is the only audience viewing great dramas and acts of courage. Such privilege demands a response to the actor. Though patients may have other confidants, none is likely to have the therapist's comprehensive appreciation of certain momentous acts. For example, years ago a patient, Michael, a novelist, informed me one day that he had just closed his secret post office box. For years this mailbox had been his method of communication in a long series of clandestine extramarital affairs. Hence, closing the box was a momentous act, and I considered it my responsibility to appreciate the great courage of his act and made a point of expressing to him my admiration for his action.

A few months later he was still tormented by recurring images and cravings for his last lover. I offered support.

> "You know, Michael, the type of passion you experienced doesn't ever evaporate quickly. Of course you're going to be revisited with longings. It's inevitable—that's part of your humanity."
>
> "Part of my weakness, you mean. I wish I were a man of steel and could put her aside for good."
>
> "We have a name for such men of steel: robots. And a

robot, thank God, is what you are not. We've talked often about your sensitivity and your creativity—these are your richest assets—that's why your writing is so powerful and that's why others are drawn to you. But these very traits have a dark side—anxiety—they make it impossible for you to live through such circumstances with equanimity."

A lovely example of a reframed comment that provided much comfort to me occurred some time ago when I expressed my disappointment at a bad review of one of my books to a friend, William Blatty, the author of *The Exorcist*. He responded in a wonderfully supportive manner, which instantaneously healed my wound. "Irv, of course you're upset by the review. Thank God for it! If you weren't so sensitive, you wouldn't be such a good writer."

All therapists will discover their own way of supporting patients. I have an indelible image in my mind of Ram Dass describing his leave-taking from a guru with whom he had studied at an ashram in India for many years. When Ram Dass lamented that he was not ready to leave because of his many flaws and imperfections, his guru rose and slowly and very solemnly circled him in a close-inspection tour, which he concluded with an official pronouncement: "I see no imperfections." I've never literally circled patients, visually inspecting them, and I never feel that the process of growth ever ends, but nonetheless this image has often guided my comments.

Support may include comments about appearance: some article of clothing, a well-rested, suntanned countenance, a new hairstyle. If a patient obsesses about physical unattractiveness I believe the human thing to do is to comment (if one feels this way) that you consider him/her to be attractive and to wonder about the origins of the myth of his/her unattractiveness.

In a story about psychotherapy in *Momma and the Meaning*

of Life, my protagonist, Dr. Ernest Lash, is cornered by an exceptionally attractive female patient, who presses him with explicit questions: "Am I appealing to men? To you? If you weren't my therapist would you respond sexually to me?" These are the ultimate nightmarish questions—the questions therapists dread above all others. It is the fear of such questions that causes many therapists to give too little of themselves. But I believe the fear is unwarranted. If you deem it in the patient's best interests, why not simply say, as my fictional character did, "If everything were different, we met in another world, I were single, I weren't your therapist, then yes, I would find you very attractive and sure would make an effort to know you better." What's the risk? In my view such candor simply increases the patient's trust in you and in the process of therapy. Of course, this does not preclude other types of inquiry about the question—about, for example, the patient's motivation or timing (the standard "Why now?" question) or inordinate preoccupation with physicality or seduction, which may be obscuring even more significant questions.

CHAPTER 6

Empathy: Looking Out the Patient's Window

It's strange how certain phrases or events lodge in one's mind and offer ongoing guidance or comfort. Decades ago I saw a patient with breast cancer, who had, throughout adolescence, been locked in a long, bitter struggle with her naysaying father. Yearning for some form of reconciliation, for a new, fresh beginning to their relationship, she looked forward to her father's driving her to college—a time when she would be alone with him for several hours. But the long-anticipated trip proved a disaster: her father behaved true to form by grousing at length about the ugly, garbage-littered creek by the side of the road. She, on the other hand, saw no litter whatsoever in the beautiful, rustic, unspoiled stream. She could find no way to respond and eventually, lapsing into silence, they spent the remainder of the trip looking away from each other.

Later, she made the same trip alone and was astounded to note that there were *two* streams—one on each side of the road. "This time I was the driver," she said sadly, "and the stream I

saw through my window on the driver's side was just as ugly
and polluted as my father had described it." But by the time
she had learned to look out her father's window, it was too
late—her father was dead and buried.

That story has remained with me, and on many occasions I
have reminded myself and my students, "Look out the other's
window. Try to see the world as your patient sees it." The
woman who told me this story died a short time later of breast
cancer, and I regret that I cannot tell her how useful her story
has been over the years, to me, my students, and many
patients.

Fifty years ago Carl Rogers identified "accurate empathy" as
one of the three essential characteristics of the effective therapist (along with "unconditional positive regard" and "genuineness") and launched the field of psychotherapy research, which
ultimately marshaled considerable evidence to support the
effectiveness of empathy.

Therapy is enhanced if the therapist enters accurately into
the patient's world. Patients profit enormously simply from the
experience of being fully seen and fully understood. Hence, it
is important for us to appreciate how our patient experiences
the past, present, and future. I make a point of repeatedly
checking out my assumptions. For example:

"Bob, when I think about your relationship to Mary,
this is what I understand. You say you are convinced that
you and she are incompatible, that you want very much
to separate from her, that you feel bored in her company
and avoid spending entire evenings with her. Yet now,
when she has made the move you wanted and has pulled
away, you once again yearn for her. I think I hear you saying that you don't want to be with her, yet you cannot

bear the idea of her not being available when you might
need her. Am I right so far?"

Accurate empathy is most important in the domain of the
immediate present—that is, the here-and-now of the therapy
hour. *Keep in mind that patients view the therapy hours very differently from therapists.* Again and again, therapists, even highly
experienced ones, are greatly surprised to rediscover this phenomenon. Not uncommonly, one of my patients begins an hour
by describing an intense emotional reaction to something that
occurred during the previous hour, and I feel baffled and cannot for the life of me imagine what it was that happened in that
hour to elicit such a powerful response.

Such divergent views between patient and therapist first
came to my attention years ago, when I was conducting
research on the experience of group members in both therapy
groups and encounter groups. I asked a great many group members to fill out a questionnaire in which they identified critical
incidents for each meeting. The rich and varied incidents
described differed greatly from their group leaders' assessments
of each meeting's critical incidents, and a similar difference
existed between members' and leaders' selection of the most
critical incidents for the entire group experience.

My next encounter with differences in patient and therapist perspectives occurred in an informal experiment, in which
a patient and I each wrote summaries of each therapy hour.
The experiment has a curious history. The patient, Ginny, was
a gifted creative writer who suffered from not only a severe
writing block, but a block in all forms of expressiveness. A
year's attendance in my therapy group was relatively unproductive: She revealed little of herself, gave little of herself to the
other members, and idealized me so greatly that any genuine

encounter was not possible. Then, when Ginny had to leave the group because of financial pressures, I proposed an unusual experiment. I offered to see her in individual therapy with the proviso that, in lieu of payment, she write a free-flowing, uncensored summary of each therapy hour expressing all the feelings and thoughts she had not verbalized during our session. I, for my part, proposed to do exactly the same and suggested we each hand in our sealed weekly reports to my secretary and that every few months we would read each other's notes.

My proposal was overdetermined. I hoped that the writing assignment might not only liberate my patient's writing, but encourage her to express herself more freely in therapy. Perhaps, I hoped, her reading my notes might improve our relationship. I intended to write uncensored notes revealing my own experiences during the hour: my pleasures, frustrations, distractions. It was possible that, if Ginny could see me more realistically, she could begin to de-idealize me and relate to me on a more human basis.

(As an aside, not germane to this discussion of empathy, I would add that this experience occurred at a time when I was attempting to develop my voice as a writer, and my offer to write in parallel with my patient had also a self-serving motive: It afforded me an unusual writing exercise and an opportunity to break my professional shackles, to liberate my voice by writing all that came to mind immediately following each hour.)

The exchange of notes every few months provided a *Rashomon*-like experience: Though we had shared the hour, we experienced and remembered it idiosyncratically. For one thing, we valued very different parts of the session. My elegant and brilliant interpretations? *She never even heard them.* Instead, she valued the small personal acts I barely noticed: my complimenting her clothing or appearance or writing, my awkward apologies for arriving a couple of minutes late, my chuckling at her satire, my teasing her when we role-played.*

All these experiences have taught me not to assume that the patient and I have the same experience during the hour. When patients discuss feelings they had the previous session, I make a point of inquiring about their experience and almost always learn something new and unexpected. Being empathic is so much a part of everyday discourse—popular singers warble platitudes about being in the other's skin, walking in the other's moccasins—that we tend to forget the complexity of the process. It is extraordinarily difficult to know really what the other feels; far too often we project our own feelings onto the other.

When teaching students about empathy, Erich Fromm often cited Terence's statement from two thousand years ago—"I am human and let nothing human be alien to me"—and urged us to be open to that part of ourselves that corresponds to any deed or fantasy offered by patients, no matter how heinous, violent, lustful, masochistic, or sadistic. If we didn't, he suggested we investigate why we have chosen to close that part of ourselves.

Of course, a knowledge of the patient's past vastly enhances your ability to look out the patient's window. If, for example, patients have suffered a long series of losses, then they will view the world through the spectacles of loss. They may be dis-

---

*Later, I used the session summaries in psychotherapy teaching and was struck by their pedagogical value. Students reported that our joint notes took on the characteristics of an epistolary novel and eventually, in 1974, the patient, Ginny Elkin (a pseudonym), and I published them under the title *Every Day Gets a Little Closer*. Twenty years later, the book was released in paperback and began a new life. In retrospect the subtitle, *A Twice-Told Therapy*, would have been more apt, but Ginny loved the old Buddy Holly song and wanted to get married to its tune.

inclined, for example, to let you matter or get too close because of fear of suffering yet another loss. Hence the investigation of the past may be important not for the sake of constructing causal chains but because it permits us to be more accurately empathic.

CHAPTER 7

Teach Empathy

Accurate empathy is an essential trait not only for therapists but for patients, *and we must help patients develop empathy for others.* Keep in mind that our patients generally come to see us because of their lack of success in developing and maintaining gratifying interpersonal relationships. Many fail to empathize with the feelings and experiences of others.

I believe that the here-and-now offers therapists a powerful way to help patients develop empathy. The strategy is straightforward: Help patients experience empathy with you, and they will automatically make the necessary extrapolations to other important figures in their lives. It is quite common for therapists to ask patients how a certain statement or action of theirs might affect others. I suggest simply that the therapist include himself in that question.

When patients venture a guess about how I feel, I generally hone in on it. If, for example, a patient interprets some gesture or comment and says, "You must be very tired of seeing me," or "I know you're sorry you ever got involved with me," or "I've got to be your most unpleasant hour of the day," I will do some reality testing and comment, "Is there a question in there for me?"

This is, of course, simple social-skills training: I urge the patient to address or question me directly, and I endeavor to answer in a manner that is direct and helpful. For example, I might respond: "You're reading me entirely wrong. I don't have any of those feelings. I've been pleased with our work. You've shown a lot of courage, you work hard, you've never missed a session, you've never been late, you've taken chances by sharing so many intimate things with me. In every way here, you do your job. But I do notice that whenever you venture a guess about how I feel about you, it often does not jibe with my inner experience, and the error is always in the same direction: You read me as caring for you much less than I do."

Another example:

> "I know you've heard this story before but . . ." (and the patient proceeded to tell a long story).
> "I'm struck by how often you say that I've heard the story before and then proceed to tell it."
> "It's a bad habit, I know. I don't understand it."
> "What's your hunch about how I feel listening to the same story over again?"
> "Must be tedious. You probably want the hour to end—you're probably checking the clock."
> "Is there a question in there for me?"
> "Well, do you?"
> "I *am* impatient hearing the same story again. I feel it

gets interposed between the two of us, as though you're not really talking to me. You were right about my checking the clock. I did—but it was with the hope that when your story ended we would still have time to make contact before the end of the session."

CHAPTER 8

Let the Patient Matter to You

It was more than thirty years ago that I heard the saddest of psychotherapy tales. I was spending a year's fellowship in London at the redoubtable Tavistock Clinic and met with a prominent British psychoanalyst and group therapist who was retiring at the age of seventy and the evening before had held the final meeting of a long-term therapy group. The members, many of whom had been in the group for more than a decade, had reflected upon the many changes they had seen in one another, and all had agreed that there was one person who had not changed whatsoever: the therapist! In fact, they said he was *exactly* the same after ten years. He then looked up at me and, tapping on his desk for emphasis, said in his most teacherly voice: "That, my boy, is good technique."

I've always been saddened as I recall this incident. It is sad to think of being together with others for so long and yet never to have let them matter enough to be influenced and changed by them. I urge you to let your patients matter to you, to let them enter your mind, influence you, change you—and not to conceal this from them.

Years ago I listened to a patient vilifying several of her friends for "sleeping around." This was typical of her: she was highly critical of everyone she described to me. I wondered aloud about the impact of her judgmentalism on her friends:

> "What do you mean?" she responded. "Does my judging others have an impact on *you*?"
>
> "I think it makes me wary of revealing too much of myself. If we were involved as friends, I'd be cautious about showing you my darker side."
>
> "Well, this issue seems pretty black-and-white to me. What's your opinion about such casual sex? Can you personally possibly imagine separating sex from love?"
>
> "Of course I can. That's part of our human nature."
>
> "That repulses me."

The hour ended on that note and for days afterward I felt unsettled by our interaction, and I began the following session by telling her that it had been very uncomfortable for me to think that she was repulsed by me. She was startled by my reaction and told me I had entirely misunderstood her: what she had meant was that she was repulsed at human nature and at her own sexual wishes, not repulsed by me or my words.

Later in the session she returned to the incident and said that though she regretted being the cause of discomfort for me, she was nonetheless moved—and pleased—at having mattered to me. The interchange dramatically catalyzed therapy: in subsequent sessions she trusted me more and took much greater risks.

Recently one of my patients sent me an E-mail:

I love you but I also hate you because you leave, not just to Argentina and New York and for all I know, to Tibet and Timbuktu, but because every week you leave, you close the door, you probably just go turn on the baseball game or check the Dow and make a cup of tea whistling a happy tune and don't think of me at all and why should you?

This statement gives voice to the great unasked question for many patients: "Do you ever think about me between sessions or do I just drop out of your life for the rest of the week?"

My experience is that often patients do not vanish from my mind for the week, and if I've had thoughts since the last session that might be helpful for them to hear, I make sure to share them.

If I feel I've made an error in the session, I believe it is always best to acknowledge it directly. Once a patient described a dream:

"I'm in my old elementary school and I speak to a little girl who is crying and has run out of her classroom. I say, 'You must remember that there are many who love you and it would be best not to run away from everyone.'"

I suggested that she was both the speaker and the little girl and that the dream paralleled and echoed the very thing we had been discussing in our last session. She responded, "Of course."

That nettled me: she characteristically failed to acknowledge my helpful comments and therefore I insisted on analyzing her comment, "Of course." Later, as I thought about this unsatisfying session, I realized the problem between us had been due largely to my stubborn determination to crack the "of course" in order to obtain full credit for my insight into the dream.

I opened the following session by acknowledging my immature behavior, and then we proceeded to have one of our most productive sessions, in which she revealed several important secrets she had long withheld. Therapist disclosure begets patient disclosure.

Patients sometimes matter enough to enter into my dreams and, if I believe that it will in some way facilitate therapy, I do not hesitate to share the dream. I once dreamed that I met a patient in an airport and attempted to give her a hug but was obstructed by the large purse she was holding. I related the dream to her and connected it to our discussion in our previous session about the "baggage" she brought into her relationship with me—that is, her strong and ambivalent feelings toward her father. She was moved by my sharing the dream and acknowledged the logic of my connecting it to her conflation of her father and me, but suggested another, cogent meaning to the dream—namely, that the dream expresses my regrets that our professional contract (symbolized by the purse, a container for money, to wit, the therapy fees) precluded a fully consummated relationship. I couldn't deny that her interpretation made compelling sense and that it reflected feelings lurking somewhere deep within me.

CHAPTER 9

Acknowledge Your Errors

It was the analyst D. W. Winnicott who once made the trenchant observation that the difference between good mothers and bad mothers is not the *commission* of errors *but what they do with them.*

I saw one patient who had left her previous therapist for what might appear a trivial reason. In their third meeting she had wept copiously and reached for the Kleenex only to find an empty box. The therapist had then begun searching his office in vain for a tissue or a handkerchief and finally scurried down the hall to the washroom to return with a handful of toilet tissue. In the following session she commented that the incident must have been embarrassing for him, whereupon he denied any embarrassment whatsoever. The more she pressed, the more he dug in and turned the questions back to why she persisted in doubting his answer. Eventually she concluded (rightly, it seemed to me) that he had not dealt with her in an authentic manner and decided that she could not trust him for the long work ahead.

An example of acknowledged error: A patient who had suffered many earlier losses and was dealing with the impending loss of her husband, who was dying of a brain tumor, once asked me whether I ever thought about her between sessions. I responded, "I often think about your situation." Wrong answer! My words outraged her. "How could you say this," she asked, "you, who were supposed to help—you, who ask me to share my innermost personal feelings. Those words reinforce my fears that I have no self—that everyone thinks about my *situation* and no one thinks about me." Later she added that not only does she have no self, but that I also avoided bringing my own self into my meetings with her.

I brooded about her words during the following week and, concluding that she was absolutely correct, began the next session by owning up to my error and by asking her to help me identify and understand my own blind spots in this matter. (Many years ago I read an article by Sándor Ferenczi, a gifted analyst, in which he reported saying to a patient, "Perhaps you can help me locate some of my own blind spots." This is another one of those phrases that have taken up lodging in my mind and that I often make use of in my clinical work.)

Together we looked at my alarm at the depth of her anguish and my deep desire to find some way, *any* way short of physical holding, to comfort her. Perhaps, I suggested, I had been backing away from her in recent sessions because of concern that I had been too seductive by promising much more relief than I would ever be able to deliver. I believed that this was the context for my impersonal statement about her "situation." It would have been so much better, I told her, to have simply been honest about my aching to console her and my confusion about how to proceed.

If you make a mistake, admit it. Any attempt at cover-up will ultimately backfire. At some level the patient will sense you are acting in bad faith, and therapy will suffer. Furthermore, an open admission of error is good model-setting for patients and another sign that they matter to you.

CHAPTER 10

Create a New Therapy
for Each Patient

There is a great paradox inherent in much contemporary psychotherapy research. Because researchers have a legitimate need to compare one form of psychotherapy treatment with some other treatment (pharmacological or another form of psychotherapy), they must offer a "standardized" therapy—that is, a uniform therapy for all the subjects in the project that can in the future be replicated by other researchers and therapists. (In other words, the same standards hold as in testing the effects of a pharmacological agent: namely, that all the subjects receive the same purity and potency of a drug and that the exact same drug will be available for future patients.) *And yet that very act of standardization renders the therapy less real and less effective.* Pair that problem with the fact that so much psychotherapy research uses inexperienced therapists or student therapists, and it is not hard to understand why such research has, at best, a most tenuous connection with reality.

Consider the task of experienced therapists. They must

establish a relationship with the patient characterized by genuineness, positive unconditional regard, and spontaneity. They
urge patients to begin each session with their "point of
urgency" (as Melanie Klein put it) and to explore with ever
greater depth their important issues as they unfold in the
moment of encounter. What issues? Perhaps some feeling
about the therapist. Or some issue that may have emerged as a
result of the previous session, or from one's dreams the night
before the session. My point is that therapy is spontaneous, the
relationship is dynamic and ever-evolving, and there is a continuous sequence of experiencing and then examining the
process.

At its very core, the flow of therapy should be spontaneous,
forever following unanticipated riverbeds; it is grotesquely distorted by being packaged into a formula that enables inexperienced, inadequately trained therapists (or computers) to
deliver a uniform course of therapy. One of the true abomina-
tions spawned by the managed-care movement is the ever
greater reliance on protocol therapy in which therapists are
required to adhere to a prescribed sequence, a schedule of topics and exercises to be followed each week.

In his autobiography, Jung describes his appreciation of the
uniqueness of each patient's inner world and language, a
uniqueness that requires the therapist to invent a new therapy
language for each patient. Perhaps I am overstating the case,
but I believe the present crisis in psychotherapy is so serious
and therapist spontaneity so endangered that a radical corrective is demanded. We need to go even further: *the therapist
must strive to create a new therapy for each patient.*

Therapists must convey to the patient that their paramount
task is to build a relationship together that will itself become
the agent of change. It is extremely difficult to teach this skill
in a crash course using a protocol. Above all, the therapist must

be prepared to go wherever the patient goes, do all that is necessary to continue building trust and safety in the relationship. I try to tailor the therapy for each patient, to find the best way to work, and I consider the process of shaping the therapy not the groundwork or prelude but the essence of the work. These remarks have relevance even for brief-therapy patients but pertain primarily to therapy with patients in a position to afford (or qualify for) open-ended therapy.

I try to avoid technique that is prefabricated and do best if I allow my choices to flow spontaneously from the demands of the immediate clinical situation. I believe "technique" is facilitative when it emanates from the therapist's unique encounter with the patient. Whenever I suggest some intervention to my supervisees they often try to cram it into the next session and it always bombs. Hence I have learned to preface my comments with: *"Do* not *try this in your next session,* but in this situation I might have said something like this. . . ." My point is that every course of therapy consists of small and large spontaneously generated responses or techniques that are impossible to program in advance.

Of course, technique has a different meaning for the novice than for the expert. One needs technique in learning to play the piano but eventually, if one is to make music, one must transcend learned technique and trust one's spontaneous moves.

For example, a patient who had suffered a series of painful losses appeared one day at her session in great despair, having just learned of her father's death. She was already so deep in grief from her husband's death a few months earlier that she could not bear to think of flying back to her parents' home for the funeral and of seeing her father's grave next to the grave of her brother, who had died at a young age. Nor, on the other hand, could she deal with the guilt of *not* attending her own father's funeral. Usually she was an extraordinarily resourceful and effective individual, who had often been critical of me and others for trying to "fix" things for her. But now she needed something from me—something tangible, something guilt-absolving. I responded by instructing her not to go to the funeral ("doctor's orders," I put it). Instead I scheduled our next meeting at the precise time of the funeral and devoted it entirely to reminiscences of her father. Two years later, when terminating therapy, she described how helpful this session had been.

Another patient felt so overwhelmed with stress in her life that during one session she could barely speak but simply hugged herself and rocked gently. I experienced a powerful urge to comfort her, to hold her and tell her that everything was going to be all right. I dismissed the notion of a hug—she had been sexually abused by a stepfather and I had to be particularly attentive to maintaining the feeling of safety of our relationship. Instead, at the end of the session, I impulsively offered to change the time of her next session to make it more convenient for her. Ordinarily she had to take off work to visit me and this one time I offered to see her before work, early in the morning.

The intervention did not provide the comfort I had hoped but still proved useful. Recall the fundamental therapy principle that all that happens is grist for the mill. In this instance the patient felt suspicious and threatened by my offer. She was convinced that I did not really want to meet with her, that our hours together were my low point of the week, and that I was changing her appointment time for my own, not her, convenience. That led us into the fertile territory of her self-contempt and the projection of her self-hatred onto me.

CHAPTER 11

The Therapeutic Act, Not
the Therapeutic Word

Take advantage of opportunities to learn from patients. Make a point of inquiring often into the patient's view of what is helpful about the therapy process. Earlier I stressed that therapists and patients do not often concur in their conclusions about the useful aspects of therapy. The patients' views of helpful events in therapy are generally relational, often involving some act of the therapist that stretched outside the frame of therapy or some graphic example of the therapist's consistency and presence. For example, one patient cited my willingness to meet with him even after he informed me by phone that he was sick with the flu. (Recently his couples therapist, fearing contagion, had cut short a session when he began sneezing and coughing.) Another patient, who had been convinced that I would ultimately abandon her because of her chronic rage, told me at the end of therapy that my single most helpful intervention was my making a rule to schedule an extra session automatically whenever she had angry outbursts toward me.

In another end-of-therapy debriefing a patient cited an incident when, in a session just before I left on a trip, she had handed me a story she had written and I had sent her a note to tell her how much I liked her writing. The letter was concrete evidence of my caring and she often turned to it for support during my absence. Checking in by phone to a highly distressed or suicidal patient takes little time and is highly meaningful to the patient. One patient, a compulsive shoplifter who had already served jail time, told me that the most important gesture in a long course of therapy was a supportive phone call I made when I was out of town during the Christmas shopping season—a time when she was often out of control. She felt she could not possibly be so ungrateful as to steal when I had gone out of my way to demonstrate my concern. If therapists have a concern about fostering dependency, they may ask the patient to participate in devising a strategy of how they can be most supported during critical periods.

On another occasion the same patient was compulsively shoplifting but had so changed her behavior that she was now stealing inexpensive items—for example, candy bars or cigarettes. Her rationale for stealing was, as always, that she needed to help balance the family budget. This belief was patently irrational: for one thing, she was wealthy (but refused to acquaint herself with her husband's holdings); furthermore, the amount she saved by stealing was insignificant.

"What can I do to help you now?" I asked. "How do we help you get past the feeling of being poor?" "We could start with you giving me some money," she said mischievously. Whereupon I took out my wallet and gave her fifty dollars in an envelope with instructions to take out of it the value of the item that she was about to steal. In other words, she was to steal from me rather than the storekeeper. The intervention permitted her to cut short the compulsive spree that had taken control of her, and a month later she returned the fifty dollars to me. From that point on we referred often to the incident whenever she used the rationalization of poverty.

A colleague told me that he had once treated a dancer who told him at the end of therapy that the most meaningful act of therapy was his attending one of her dance recitals. Another patient, at the end of therapy, cited my willingness to perform aura therapy. A believer in New Age concepts, she entered my office one day convinced that she was feeling ill because of a rupture in her aura. She lay down on my carpet and I followed her instructions and attempted to heal the rupture by passing my hands from head to toe a few inches above her body. I had often expressed skepticism about various New Age approaches and she regarded my agreeing to accede to her request as a sign of loving respect.

CHAPTER 12

Engage in Personal Therapy

To my mind, personal psychotherapy is, by far, the most important part of psychotherapy training. Question: What is the therapist's most valuable instrument? Answer (and no one misses this one): the therapist's own self. I will discuss the rationale and the technique of the therapist's use of self from many perspectives throughout this text. Let me begin by simply stating that therapists must show the way to patients by personal modeling. We must demonstrate our willingness to enter into a deep intimacy with our patient, a process that requires us to be adept at mining the best source of reliable data about our patient—our own feelings.

Therapists must be familiar with their own dark side and be able to empathize with all human wishes and impulses. A personal therapy experience permits the student therapist to experience many aspects of the therapeutic process from the patient's seat: the tendency to idealize the therapist, the yearning for dependency, the gratitude toward a caring and attentive listener, the power granted to the therapist. Young therapists must work through their own neurotic issues; they must learn to accept feedback, discover their own blind spots, and see themselves as others see them; they must appreciate their impact upon others and learn how to provide accurate feedback. Lastly, psychotherapy is a psychologically demanding enterprise, and therapists must develop the awareness and inner strength to cope with the many occupational hazards inherent in it.

Many training programs insist that students have a course of personal psychotherapy: for example, some California graduate psychology schools now require sixteen to thirty hours of individual therapy. That's a good start—but only a start. Self-exploration is a lifelong process, and I recommend that therapy be as deep and prolonged as possible—and that the therapist enter therapy at many different stages of life.

My own odyssey of therapy, over my forty-five-year career, is as follows: a 750-hour, five-time-a-week orthodox Freudian psychoanalysis in my psychiatric residency (with a training analyst in the conservative Baltimore Washington School), a year's analysis with Charles Rycroft (an analyst in the "middle school" of the British Psychoanalytic Institute), two years with Pat Baumgartner (a gestalt therapist), three years of psychotherapy with Rollo May (an interpersonally and existentially oriented analyst of the William Alanson White Institute), and numerous briefer stints with therapists from a variety of disciplines, including behavioral therapy, bioenergetics, Rolfing, marital-couples work, an ongoing ten-year (at this writing) leaderless support group of male therapists, and, in the 1960s, encounter groups of a whole rainbow of flavors, including a nude marathon group.

Note two aspects of this list. First, the *diversity of approaches.* It is important for the young therapist to avoid sectarianism and to gain an appreciation of the strengths of all the varying therapeutic approaches. Though students may have to sacrifice the certainty that accompanies orthodoxy, they obtain something quite precious—a greater appreciation of the complexity and uncertainty underlying the therapeutic enterprise.

I believe there is no better way to learn about a psychotherapy approach than to enter into it as a patient. Hence, I have considered a period of discomfort in my life as an educational opportunity to explore what various approaches have to offer. Of course, the particular type of discomfort has to fit the method; for example, behavioral therapy is best suited to treat a discrete symptom—hence I turned to a behaviorist to help with insomnia, which occurred when I traveled to give lectures or workshops.

Secondly, I entered therapy *at many different stages of my life*. Despite an excellent and extensive course of therapy at the onset of one's career, an entirely different set of issues may arrive at different junctures of the life cycle. It was only when I began working extensively with dying patients (in my fourth decade) that I experienced considerable explicit death anxiety. No one enjoys anxiety—and certainly not I—but I welcomed the opportunity to explore this inner domain with a good therapist. Furthermore, at the time I was engaged in writing a textbook, *Existential Psychotherapy*, and I knew that deep personal exploration would broaden my knowledge of existential issues. And so I began a fruitful and enlightening course of therapy with Rollo May.

Many training programs offer, as part of the curriculum, an experiential training group—that is, a group that focuses on its own process. These groups have much to teach, though they are often anxiety-provoking for participants (and not easy for the leaders, either—they have to get a handle on the student members' competitiveness and their complex relationships outside the group). I believe that the young psychotherapist generally profits even more from a "stranger" experiential group or, better yet, an ongoing high-functioning psychotherapy group. Only by being a member of a group can one truly appreciate such phenomena as group pressure, the relief of catharsis, the power inherent in the group-leader role, the painful but valuable process of obtaining valid feedback about one's interpersonal presentation. Last, if you are fortunate enough to be in a cohesive, hardworking group, I assure you that you will never forget it and will endeavor to provide such a therapeutic group experience for your future patients.

CHAPTER 13

The Therapist Has Many Patients; The Patient, One Therapist

There are times when my patients lament the inequality of the psychotherapy situation. They think about me far more than I think about them. I loom far larger in their lives than they do in mine. If patients could ask any question they wished, I am certain that, for many, that question would be: Do you ever think about me?

There are many ways to address this situation. For one, keep in mind that, though the inequality may be irritating for many patients, it is at the same time important and necessary. We *want* to loom large in the patient's mind. Freud once pointed out that it is important for the therapist to loom so large in the patient's mind that the interactions between the patient and therapist begin to influence the course of the patient's symptomatology (that is, the psychoneurosis becomes gradually replaced by a transference neurosis). We want the therapy hour to be one of the most important events in the patient's life.

Though it is not our goal to do away with all powerful feelings toward the therapist, there are times when the transference feelings are too dysphoric, times when the patient is so tormented by feelings about the therapist that some decompression is necessary. I am apt to enhance reality testing by commenting upon the inherent cruelty of the therapy situation—the basic nature of the arrangement dictates that the patient think more about the therapist than vice versa: *The patient has only one therapist while the therapist has many patients.* Often I find the teacher analogy useful, and point out that the teacher has many students but the students have only one teacher and, *of course*, students think more about their teacher than she about them. If the patient has had teaching experience, this may be particularly relevant. Other relevant professions—for example, physician, nurse, supervisor—also may be cited.

Another aid I have often used is to refer to my personal experience as a psychotherapy patient by saying something like: "I know it feels unfair and unequal for you to be thinking of me more than I of you, for you to be carrying on long conversations with me between sessions, knowing that I do not similarly speak in fantasy to you. But that's simply the nature of the process. I had exactly the same experience during my own time in therapy, when I sat in the patient's chair and yearned to have my therapist think more about me."

CHAPTER 14

The Here-and-Now—Use It, Use It, Use It

The here-and-now is the major source of therapeutic power, the pay dirt of therapy, the therapist's (and hence the patient's) best friend. So vital for effective therapy is the here-and-now that I shall discuss it more extensively than any other topic in this text.

The here-and-now refers to the immediate events of the therapeutic hour, to what is happening *here* (in this office, in this relationship, in the *in-betweenness*—the space between me and you) and *now*, in this immediate hour. It is basically an ahistoric approach and *de-emphasizes* (but does *not negate the importance of*) the patient's historical past or events of his or her outside life.

CHAPTER 15

Why Use the Here-and-Now?

The rationale for using the here-and-now rests upon a couple of basic assumptions: (1) the importance of interpersonal relationships and (2) the idea of therapy as a social microcosm.

To the social scientist and the contemporary therapist, interpersonal relationships are so obviously and monumentally important that to belabor the issue is to run the risk of preaching to the converted. Suffice it to say that regardless of our professional perspective—whether we study our nonhuman primate relatives, primitive cultures, the individual's developmental history, or current life patterns—it is apparent that we are intrinsically social creatures. Throughout life, our surrounding interpersonal environment—peers, friends, teachers, as well as family—has enormous influence over the kind of individual we become. Our self-image is formulated to a large degree upon the reflected appraisals we perceive in the eyes of the important figures in our life.

Furthermore the great majority of individuals seeking therapy have fundamental problems in their relationships; by and large people fall into despair because of their inability to form and maintain enduring and gratifying interpersonal relationships. Psychotherapy based on the interpersonal model is directed toward removing the obstacles to satisfying relationships.

The second postulate—that therapy is a social microcosm—means that eventually (provided we do not structure it too heavily) *the interpersonal problems of the patient will manifest themselves in the here-and-now of the therapy relationship*. If, in his or her life, the patient is demanding or fearful or arrogant or self-effacing or seductive or controlling or judgmental or maladaptive interpersonally in any other way, then *these traits will enter into the patient's relationship with the therapist*. Again, this approach is basically ahistoric: There is little need of extensive history-taking to apprehend the nature of maladaptive patterns *because they will soon enough be displayed in living color in the here-and-now of the therapy hour*.

To summarize, the rationale for using the here-and-now is that human problems are largely relational and that an individual's interpersonal problems will ultimately be manifested in the here-and-now of the therapy encounter.

CHAPTER 16

Using the Here-and-Now—
Grow Rabbit Ears

One of the first steps in therapy is to identify the here-and-now equivalents of your patient's interpersonal problems. An essential part of your education is to learn to focus on the here-and-now. *You must develop here-and-now rabbit ears.* The everyday events of each therapy hour are rich with data: consider how patients greet you, take a seat, inspect or fail to inspect their surroundings, begin and end the session, recount their history, relate to you.

My office is in a separate cottage about a hundred feet down a winding garden path from my house. Since every patient walks down the same path, I have over the years accumulated much comparison data. Most patients comment about the garden—the profusion of fleecy lavender blossoms; the sweet, heavy wisteria fragrance; the riot of purple, pink, coral, and crimson—but some do not. One man never failed to make some negative comment: the mud on the path, the need for guardrails in the rain, or the sound of leaf-blowers from a neighboring house. I give all patients the same directions to my office for their first visit: Drive down X street a half mile past XX Road, make a right turn at XXX Avenue, at which there's a sign for Fresca (a local attractive restaurant) on the corner. Some patients comment on the directions, some do not. One particular patient (the same one who complained about the muddy path) confronted me in an early session: "How come you chose Fresca as your landmark rather than Taco Tio?" (Taco Tio is a Mexican fast-food eyesore on the opposite corner.)

To grow rabbit ears, keep in mind this principle: *One stimulus, many reactions*. If individuals are exposed to a common complex stimulus, they are likely to have very different responses. This phenomenon is particularly evident in group therapy, in which group members simultaneously experience the same stimulus—for example, a member's weeping, or late arrival, or confrontation with the therapist—and yet each of them has a very different response to the event.

Why does that happen? There is only one possible explanation: *Each individual has a different internal world and the stimulus has a different meaning to each*. In individual therapy the same principle obtains, only the events occur sequentially rather than simultaneously (that is, many patients of one therapist are, over time, exposed to the same stimulus. Therapy is like a living Rorschach test—patients project onto it perceptions, attitudes, and meanings from their own unconscious).

I develop certain baseline expectations because all my patients encounter the same person (assuming I am reasonably stable), receive the same directions to my office, walk down the same path to get there, enter the same room with the same furnishings. Thus the patient's idiosyncratic response is deeply informative—a *via regia* permitting you to understand the patient's inner world.

When the latch on my screen door was broken, preventing the door from closing snugly, my patients responded in a number of ways. One patient invariably spent much time fiddling with it and each week apologized for it as though she had broken it. Many ignored it, while others never failed to point out the defect and suggest I should get it fixed. Some wondered why I delayed so long.

Even the banal Kleenex box may be a rich source of data. One patient apologized if she moved the box slightly when extracting a tissue. Another refused to take the last tissue in the box. Another wouldn't let me hand her one, saying she could do it herself. Once, when I had failed to replace an empty box, a patient joked about it for weeks ("So you remembered this time." Or, "A new box! You must be expecting a heavy session today."). Another brought me a present of two boxes of Kleenex.

Most of my patients have read some of my books, and their responses to my writing constitute a rich source of material. Some are intimidated by my having written so much. Some express concern that they will not prove interesting to me. One patient told me that he read a book of mine in snatches in the bookstore and didn't want to buy it, since he had "already given a donation at the office." Others, who make the assumption of an economy of scarcity, hate the books because my descriptions of close relationships to other patients suggest that there will be little love left for them.

In addition to responses to office surroundings, therapists have a variety of other standard reference points (for example, beginnings and endings of hours, bill payments) that generate comparative data. And then of course there is that most elegant and complex instrument of all—the Stradivarius of psychotherapy practice—the therapist's own self. I shall have much more to say about the use and care of this instrument.

CHAPTER 17

Search for Here-and-Now Equivalents

What should the therapist do when a patient brings up an issue involving some unhappy interaction with another person? Generally therapists explore the situation at great depth and try to help the patient understand his/her role in the transaction, explore options for alternative behaviors, investigate unconscious motivation, guess at the motivations of the other person, and search for patterns—that is, similar situations that the patient has created in the past. This time-honored strategy has limitations: not only is the work apt to be intellectualized but all too often it is based on inaccurate data suppled by the patient.

The here-and-now offers a far better way to work. The general strategy is to find a *here-and-now equivalent* of the dysfunctional interaction. Once this is done, the work becomes much more accurate and immediate. Some examples:

Keith and permanent grudges. Keith, a long-term patient and a practicing psychotherapist, reported a highly vitriolic interaction with his adult son. The son, for the first time, had decided to make the arrangements for the family's annual fishing and camping trip. Though pleased at his son's coming of age and at being relieved of the burden, Keith could not relinquish control, and when he attempted to override his son's planning by forcefully insisting upon a slightly earlier date and different locale, his son exploded, calling his father intrusive and controlling. Keith was devastated and absolutely convinced that he had permanently lost his son's love and respect.

What are my tasks in this situation? A long-range task, to which we would return in the future, was to explore Keith's inability to relinquish control. A more immediate task was to offer some immediate comfort and assist Keith to reestablish equilibrium. I sought to help Keith gain perspective so that he could understand that this contretemps was but one fleeting episode against the horizon of a lifetime of loving interactions with his son. I deemed it inefficient for me to analyze in great and endless depth this episode between Keith and his son, whom I had never met and whose true feelings I could only surmise. Far better, I thought, to identify and work through a here-and-now equivalent of the unsettling event.

But what here-and-now event? That's where rabbit ears are needed. As it happened, I had recently referred to Keith a patient who, after a couple of sessions with him, did not return. Keith had experienced great anxiety about losing this patient and agonized for a long time before "confessing" it in the previous session. Keith was convinced that I would judge him harshly, that I would not forgive him for failing, and that I would never again refer another patient to him. Note the symbolic equivalence of these two events—in each one, Keith presumed that a single act would forever blemish him in the eyes of someone he treasured.

I chose to pursue the here-and-now episode because of its greater immediacy and accuracy. I was the subject of Keith's apprehension and could access my own feelings rather than be limited to conjecture about how his son felt. I told him that he was misreading me entirely, that I had no doubts about his sensitivity and compassion and was certain he did excellent clinical work. It was unthinkable for me to ignore all my long experience with him on the basis of this one episode, and I said that I would refer him other patients in the future. In the final analysis I feel certain that this here-and-now therapeutic work was far more powerful than a "then-and-there" investigation of the crisis with his son and that he would remember our encounter long after he forgot any intellectual analysis of the episode with his son.

Alice and crudity. Alice, a sixty-year-old widow desperately searching for another husband, complained of a series of failed relationships with men who often vanished without explanation from her life. In our third month of therapy she took a cruise with her latest beau, Morris, who expressed his chagrin at her haggling over prices, shamelessly pushing her way to the front of lines, and sprinting for the best seats in tour buses. After their trip Morris disappeared and refused to return her calls.

Rather than embark on an analysis of her relationship with Morris, I turned to my own relationship with Alice. I was aware that I, too, wanted out and had pleasurable fantasies in which she announced she had decided to terminate. Even though she brashly (and successfully) negotiated a considerably lower therapy fee, she continued to tell me how unfair it was that I should charge her so much. She never failed to make some comment on the fee—about whether I had earned it that day, or about my unwillingness to give her an even lower senior-citizen fee. Moreover, she pressed for extra time by bringing up urgent issues just as the hour was ending or giving me items to read ("on your own time," as she put it)—her dream journal; articles on widowhood, journaling therapy, or the fallacy of Freud's beliefs. Overall, she was without delicacy and, just as she had done with Morris, turned our relationship into something crude. I knew that this here-and-now reality was where we needed to work, and the gentle exploration of how she had coarsened her relationship with me proved so useful that months later some very astonished elderly gentlemen received her phone calls of apology.

Mildred and the lack of presence. Mildred had been abused sexually as a child and had such difficulty in her physical relationship with her husband that her marriage was in jeopardy. As soon as her husband touched her sexually she began to reexperience traumatic events from her past. This paradigm made it very difficult to work on her relationship to her husband because it demanded that she first be liberated from the past—a daunting process.

As I examined the here-and-now relationship between the two of us I could appreciate many similarities between the way she related to me and the way she related to her husband. I often felt ignored in the sessions. Though she was an engaging storyteller and had the capacity to entertain me at great length, I found it difficult to be "present" with her—that is, linked, engaged, close to her, with some sense of mutuality. She rambled, never asked me about myself, appeared to have little sense or curiosity about my experience in the hour, was never "there" relating to me. Gradually, as I persisted in focusing on the "in-betweenness" of our relationship and the extent of her absence and how shut out I felt by her, Mildred began to appreciate the extent to which she exiled her husband, and one day she started a session by saying, "For some reason, I'm not sure why, I've just made a great discovery: I never look my husband in the eyes when we have sex."

Albert and swallowed rage. Albert, who commuted over an hour to my office, had often experienced panic at times when he felt he had been exploited. He knew he was suffused with anger but could find no way to express it. In one session he described a frustrating encounter with a girlfriend who, in his view, was obviously jerking him around, yet he was paralyzed with fear about confronting her. The session felt repetitious to me; we had spent considerable time in many sessions discussing the same material and I always felt I had offered him little help. I could sense his frustration with me: he implied that he had spoken to many friends who had covered all the same bases I had and had ultimately advised him to tell her off or get out of the relationship. I tried to speak for him:

> "Albert, let me see if I can guess at what you might be experiencing in this session. You travel an hour to see me and you pay me a good deal of money. Yet we seem to be repeating ourselves. You feel I don't give you much of value. I say the same things as your friends, who give it to you free. You have got to be disappointed in me, even feeling ripped off and angry at me for giving you so little."

He gave a thin smile and acknowledged that my assessment was fairly accurate. I was pretty close. I asked him to repeat it in his own words. He did that with some trepidation, and I responded that, though I couldn't be happy with not having given him what he wanted, I liked very much his stating these things directly to me: It felt better to be straighter with each other, and he had been indirectly conveying these sentiments anyway. The whole interchange proved useful to Albert. His feelings toward me were an analog of his feelings toward his girlfriend, and the experience of expressing them without a calamitous outcome was powerfully instructive.

CHAPTER 18

Working Through Issues in the Here-and-Now

S o far we have considered how to recognize patients' major problems in the here-and-now. But once that is accomplished, how then do we proceed? How can we use these here-and-now observations in the work of therapy?

Example. Return to the scene I described earlier—the screen door with the faulty latch, and my patient who fiddled with it every week and always apologized, too many times, for not being able to close the door.

> "Nancy," I said, "I'm curious about your apologizing to me. It's as though my broken door, and my laxity in getting it fixed, is somehow your fault."
> "You're right. I know that. And yet I keep on doing it."
> "Any hunches about why?"
> "I think it's got to do with how important you are and

how important therapy is to me and my wanting to make sure I don't offend you in any way."

"Nancy, can you take a guess about how I feel every time you apologize?"

"It's probably irritating for you."

I nod. "I can't deny it. But you're quick to say that—as though it is a familiar experience to you. Is there a history to this?"

"I've heard it before, many times," she says. "I can tell you it drives my husband crazy. I know I irritate a lot of people and yet I keep doing it."

"So, in the guise of apologizing and being polite, you end up irritating others. Moreover, even though you know that, you still have difficulty in stopping. There must be some kind of payoff for you. I wonder, what is it?"

That interview and subsequent sessions then took off in a number of fruitful directions, particularly in the area of her rage toward everyone—her husband, parents, children, and me. Fastidious in her habits, she revealed how unnerved the faulty screen door made her. And not only the door, but also my cluttered desk, heaped high with untidy stacks of books. She also stated how very impatient she was with me for not working faster with her.

Example. Several months into therapy, Louise, a patient who was highly critical of me—of the office furnishings, the poor color scheme, the general untidiness of my desk, my clothing, the informality and incompleteness of my bills—told me about a new romantic relationship she had formed. During the course of her account she remarked:

"Well, grudgingly, I have to admit I'm doing better."

"I'm struck by your word 'grudgingly.' Why 'grudgingly'? It seems hard for you to say positive things about me and about our work together. What do you know about that?"

No answer. Louise silently shook her head.

"Just think out loud, Louise, anything that comes to mind."

"Well, you'll get a swelled head. Can't have that."

"Keep going."

"You'll win. I'll lose."

"Win and lose? We're in a battle? And what's the battle about? And the underlying war?"

"Don't know, just a part of me that's always been there, always mocking people, looking for their bad side, seeing them sitting on a pile of their own shit."

"And with me? I'm thinking of how critical you are of my office. And of the path as well. You never fail to mention the mud but never the flowers blossoming."

"Happens with my boyfriend all the time—he'll bring me presents and I can't help focusing on how little care he has taken with the wrapping. We got in a fight last week when he baked me a loaf of bread and I made a teasing comment on the slightly burnt corner of the crust."

"You always give that side of you a voice and you keep the other side mute—the side that appreciates his making you bread, the side that likes and values me. Louise, go back to the beginning of this discussion—your comment about 'grudgingly' admitting you are better. Tell me, what would it be like if you were to unfetter the positive part of you and speak straight out, without the 'grudgingly'?"

"I see sharks circling."

"Just think of speaking to me. What do you imagine?"

"Kissing you on the lips."

For several sessions thereafter we explored her fears of closeness, of wanting too much, of unfilled, insatiable yearnings, of her love for her father, and her fears that I would bolt if I really knew how much she wanted from me. Note in this vignette that I drew upon incidents that had occurred in the past, earlier in our therapy. Here-and-now work is not strictly ahistoric, since it may include any events that have occurred throughout one's relationship with the patient. As Sartre put it, "Introspection is always retrospection."

CHAPTER 19

The Here-and-Now
Energizes Therapy

Work in the here-and-now is always more exciting than work with a more abstract or historical focus. This is particularly evident in group therapy. Consider, for example, an historical episode in group work. In 1946, the state of Connecticut sponsored a workshop to deal with racial tensions in the workplace. Small groups led by the eminent psychologist Kurt Lewin and a team of social psychologists engaged in a discussion of the "back home" problems brought up by the participants. The leaders and observers of the groups (without the group members) held nightly post-group meetings in which they discussed not only the content, but also the "process" of the sessions. (*Nota bene*: The content refers to the actual words and concepts expressed. The "process" refers to *the* nature of the relationship between the individuals who express the words and concepts.)

News spread about these evening staff meetings, and two days later the members of the groups asked to attend. After much hesitation (such a procedure was entirely novel) approval was granted, and the group members observed themselves being discussed by the leaders and researchers.

There are several published accounts of this momentous session at which the importance of the here-and-now was discovered. All agree that the meeting was electrifying; members were fascinated by hearing themselves and their behavior discussed. Soon they could stay silent no longer and interjected such comments as "No, that wasn't what I said," or "how I said it," or "what I meant." The social scientists realized that they had stumbled onto an important axiom for education (and for therapy as well): namely that we learn best about ourselves and our behavior through personal participation in interaction combined with observation and analysis of that interaction.

In group therapy the difference between a group discussing "back home" problems of the members and a group engaged in the here-and-now—that is, a discussion of their own process—is very evident: The here-and-now group is energized, members are engaged, and they will always, if questioned (either through interviews or research instruments), remark that the group comes alive when it focuses on process.

In the two-week group laboratories held for decades at Bethel, Maine, it was soon evident to all that the power and allure of process groups—first called sensitivity-training groups (that is, interpersonal sensitivity) and later "T-groups" (training) and still later "encounter groups" (Carl Rogers's term)—immediately dwarfed other groups the laboratory offered (for example, theory groups, application groups, or problem-solving groups) in terms of members' interest and enthusiasm. In fact, it was often said that the T-groups "ate up the rest of the laboratory." People want to interact with others, are excited by giving and receiving direct feedback, yearn to learn how they are perceived by others, want to slough off their facades and become intimate.

Many years ago, when I was attempting to develop a more effective mode to lead brief-therapy groups on the acute inpatient ward, I visited dozens of groups in hospitals throughout the country and found every group to be ineffective—and for precisely the same reason. Each group meeting used a "take-turns" or "check-in" format consisting of members' sequentially discussing some then-and-there event—for example, hallucinatory experiences or past suicidal inclinations or the reasons for their hospitalization—while the other members listened silently and often disinterestedly. I ultimately formulated, in a text on inpatient group therapy, a here-and-now approach for such acutely disturbed patients, which, I believe, vastly increased the degree of member engagement.

The same observation holds for individual therapy. Therapy is invariably energized when it focuses on the relationship between therapist and patient. *Every Day Gets a Little Closer* describes an experiment in which a patient and I each wrote summaries of the therapy hour. It was striking that whenever we read and discussed each other's observations—that is, whenever we focused on the here-and-now—the ensuing therapy sessions came alive.

CHAPTER 20

Use Your Own Feelings as Data

One of our major tasks in therapy is to pay attention to our immediate feelings—they represent precious data. If in the session you feel bored or irritated, confused, sexually aroused, or shut out by your patient, then regard that as valuable information. This is precisely why I so emphasize personal therapy for therapists. If you develop a deep knowledge of yourself, eliminate the majority of your blind spots, and have a good base of patient experience, you will begin to know how much of the boredom or confusion is yours and how much is evoked by the patient. It is important to make that distinction, because if it is the patient who evokes your boredom in the therapy hour, then we may confidently assume that he is boring to others in other settings.

So rather than be dismayed at boredom, welcome it and search for a way to turn it to therapeutic advantage. When did it begin? What exactly does the patient do that bores you? When I encounter boredom I might say something like this:

"Mary, let me tell you something. For the last several minutes I notice that I've been feeling disconnected from you, somewhat distanced. I'm not sure why, but I know I'm feeling different now than at the beginning of the session, when you were describing your feelings of not having gotten what you wanted from me, or last session, when you spoke more from the heart. I wonder, what is your level of connection to me today? Is your feeling similar to mine? Let's try to understand what's happening."

Some years ago I treated Martin, a successful merchant, who had to take a business trip on the day of therapy and asked me to reschedule his hour to another day in the week. I couldn't arrange this without inconveniencing my schedule and told Martin we'd have to miss the session and meet at our regular hour the following week. But later, as I thought about it, I realized I would not have hesitated to rearrange my schedule for any of my other patients.

Why couldn't I do this for Martin? It was because I did not look forward to seeing him. There was something about his mean-spiritedness that had worn me down. He was unceasingly critical of me, my office furniture, the lack of parking, my secretary, my fee, and generally began sessions by referring to my errors of the previous week.

My feeling worn down by Martin had vast implications. He had initially entered therapy because of a series of failed relationships with women, none of whom, he thought, had ever given him enough—none was sufficiently forthcoming with her proper share of restaurant or grocery bills or birthday gifts equivalent in value to the ones he had given to them (his income, mind you, was several times greater than theirs). When they took trips together, he insisted that they each put the same amount of cash into a "travel jar," and all traveling expenses, including gasoline, parking, car maintenance, tips, even newspapers, be paid for out of travel-jar cash. Furthermore, he groused often because his girlfriends did not do their full share of driving, trip planning, or map reading. Eventually Martin's lack of generosity, his obsession with absolute fairness, and his relentless criticism wore out the women in his life. And he was doing exactly the same to me! It was a good example of a self-fulfilling prophecy—he so dreaded being uncared for that his behavior brought that very thing to pass. It was my recognition of this process that permitted me to avoid responding critically (that is, take it personally) but to realize this was a pattern that he had repeated many times and that he, at bottom, wanted to change.

CHAPTER 21

Frame Here-and-Now Comments Carefully

Commentary on the here-and-now is a unique aspect of the therapeutic relationship. There are few human situations in which we are permitted, let alone *encouraged*, to comment upon the immediate behavior of the other. It feels liberating, even exhilarating—that is precisely why the encounter-group experience was so compelling. But it also feels risky, since we are not accustomed to giving and receiving feedback.

Therapists must learn to package their comments in ways that feel caring and acceptable to patients. Consider the feedback about boredom I gave in the last tip: I avoided using the word "boring" to my patient; it is not a productive word; it feels like an accusation, and may (or should) elicit some spoken or unspoken sentiment such as, "I'm not paying you to be entertained."

It is far preferable to employ terms like "distanced,"

"shut out," or "disconnected"; they give voice to your wish to be closer, more connected, and more engaged, and it is difficult for our clients to take umbrage at that. In other words, talk about how *you feel,* not about what the patient is doing.

CHAPTER 22

All Is Grist for
the Here-and-Now Mill

Everything that happens in the here-and-now is grist for the therapy mill. Sometimes it is best to offer commentary at the moment; other times it is best simply to store the incident and return to it later. If, for example, a patient weeps in anguish, it is best to store a here-and-now inquiry until some other time when one can return to the incident and make a comment to this effect: "Tom, I'd like to return to last week. Something unusual happened: You trusted me with a lot more of your feelings and wept deeply, for the first time, in front of me. Tell me, what was that like for you? How did it feel to let down barriers here? To allow me to see your tears?"

Remember, patients don't just cry or display feelings in a vacuum—they do so *in your presence,* and it is a here-and-now exploration that allows one to grasp the full meaning of the expression of feelings.

Or consider a patient who may have been very shaken during a session and, uncharacteristically, asks for a hug at the end. If I feel it is the right thing to do, I hug the patient but never fail at some point, generally in the following session, to return to the request and the hug. Keep in mind that effective therapy consists of an alternating sequence: *evocation and experiencing* of affect followed by *analysis and integration* of affect. How long one waits until one initiates an analysis of the affective event is a function of clinical experience. Often, when there is deep feeling involved—anguish, grief, anger, love—it is best to wait until the feeling simmers down and defensiveness diminishes. (See chapter 40, "Feedback: Strike When the Iron Is Cold.")

Jane was an angry, deeply demoralized woman who after several months developed enough trust in me to reveal the depth of her despair. Again and again I was so moved that I sought to offer her some comfort. But I never succeeded. Every time I tried I got bitten. But she was so brittle and so hypersensitive to perceived criticism that I waited for many weeks before I shared that observation.

Everything—especially episodes containing heightened emotion—is grist for the mill. Many unexpected events or reactions occur in therapy: Therapists may receive angry E-mail or calls from patients, they may not be able to offer the comfort desired by the patient, they may be deemed omniscient, they are never questioned, or always challenged, they may be late, make an error in billing, even schedule two patients for the same hour. Though I feel uncomfortable going through some of these experiences, I also feel confident that, if I address them properly, I can turn them into something useful in the therapeutic work.

CHAPTER 23

Check into the Here-and-Now Each Hour

I make an effort to inquire about the here-and-now at each session even if it has been productive and nonproblematic. I always say toward the end of the hour: "Let's take a minute to look at how you and I are doing today." Or, "Any feelings about the way we are working and relating?" Or, "Before we stop, shall we take a look at what's going on in this space between us?" Or if I perceive difficulties, I might say something like: "Before we stop, let's check into our relationship today. You've talked about feeling miles away from me at times, and at other times very close. What about today? How much distance between us today?" Depending on the answer, I might proceed to explore any barriers in the relationship or unspoken feelings about me.

I begin this pattern even in the very first hour, before a great deal of history has been built into the relationship. In fact, it is particularly important to start setting norms in the early sessions. In the initial session, I make certain to inquire about how patients chose to come to me. If they've been referred by someone, a colleague or friend, I want to know what they were told about me, what their expectations were, and then how their experience of me even in this first session has matched those expectations. I generally say something to this effect: "The initial session is a two-way interview. I interview you but it is also an opportunity for you to size me up and develop opinions about how it would be to work with me." This makes eminently good sense, and the patient usually nods at this. Then I always follow up with: "Could we take a look at what you've come up with so far?"

Many of my patients come to me after having read one of my books and, consequently, it is a part of the here-and-now to inquire about that. "What specifically was there about this book that brought you to me? How does the reality of seeing me match those expectations? Any concerns about a therapist who is also a writer? What questions do you wish to ask me about that?"

Ever since I wrote about patients' stories in a book (*Love's Executioner*) many years ago, I assumed that new patients consulting me might be wary of being written about. Hence I've reassured patients about confidentiality and assured them that I've never written about patients without first obtaining permission and without using deep identity disguise. But in time I have observed that patients' concerns were quite different—in general they were less concerned with being written about than with not being interesting enough to be selected.

CHAPTER 24

What Lies Have You Told Me?

Often during the course of therapy patients may describe examples of deception in their life—some incident when they have either concealed or distorted information about themselves. Using here-and-now rabbit ears, I find such an admission an excellent opportunity to inquire about what lies they have told me during the course of therapy. There is always some concealment, some information withheld because of shame, because of some particular way they wish me to regard them. A discussion of such concealments almost invariably provokes a fruitful discussion in therapy—often a review of the history of the therapy relationship and an opportunity to rework and fine-tune not only the relationship but other important themes that have previously emerged in therapy.

The general rabbit-ears strategy is simply to scan all material in the session for here-and-now implications and, whenever possible, to take the opportunity to swing into an examination of the therapy relationship.

CHAPTER 25

Blank Screen? Forget It! Be Real

The first model posited of the ideal therapist-patient relationship was the now superannuated "blank screen," in which the therapist remained neutral and more or less anonymous in the hopes that patients would project onto this blank screen major transference distortions. Once the transference (the living manifestation of earlier parental relationships) was available for study in the analysis, the therapist might more accurately reconstruct the early life of the patient. If the therapist were to manifest him-/herself as a distinct individual, it would be more difficult (so it was thought) for the projection to take place.

But forget the blank screen! It is not now, nor was it ever, a good model for effective therapy. The idea of using current distortions to re-create the past was part of an old, now abandoned, vision of the therapist as archaeologist, patiently scraping off the dust of decades to understand (and thus, in some mysterious manner, undo) the original trauma. It is a far better model to think of *understanding the past in order to apprehend the present therapist-patient relationship.* But neither of these considerations merits the sacrifice of an authentic human encounter in psychotherapy.

Did Freud himself generally follow the blank-screen model? Often, perhaps generally, not. We know this from reading his accounts of therapy (see, for example, the descriptions of therapy in *Studies in Hysteria*) or his analysands' descriptions of their analysis with Freud.

Think of Freud offering his patient a "celebratory" or "victory" cigar after making a particularly trenchant interpretation. Think of him stopping patients from rushing on to other topics and instead slowing them down to bask with him in the afterglow of an enlightening insight. The psychiatrist Roy Grinker described to me an incident in his analysis with Freud in which Freud's dog, who always attended the therapy, walked over to the door in the midst of a session. Freud rose and let the dog out. A few minutes later the dog scratched on the door for reentry and Freud rose, opened the door, and said, "You see, he couldn't stand listening to all that resistance garbage. Now he is coming back to give you a second chance."

In the case histories in *Studies in Hysteria* Freud entered personally and boldly into the lives of his patients. He made strong suggestions to them, he intervened on their behalf with family members, he contrived to attend social functions to see his patients in other settings, he instructed a patient to visit the cemetery and meditate upon the tombstone of a dead sibling.

The early blank-screen model got reinforcement from an unexpected source in the 1950s, when Carl Rogers's model of nondirective therapy instructed therapists to offer minimal direction, often limiting interventions to the echoing of the patient's last phrase. As Carl Rogers matured as a therapist he soon totally abandoned this unengaged stance with the "last-line" interview technique in favor of a far more humanistic interactive style. Nonetheless, jokes, parodies, and misunderstandings of the nondirective approach hounded him till the end of his life.

In group therapy it is exceedingly evident that one of the tasks of the group therapist is to demonstrate behavior that the group members gradually model themselves after. It is the same, though less dramatic, in individual therapy. The psychotherapy outcome literature heavily supports the view that therapist disclosure begets client disclosure.

I have long been fascinated with therapist transparency and have experimented with self-disclosure in many different formats. Perhaps my interest has its roots in my group-therapy experience, in which the demands on the therapist to be transparent are especially great. Group therapists have a particularly complex set of tasks because they must attend to not only the needs of each individual patient in the group, but to the creation and maintenance of the enveloping social system—the small group. Hence, they must attend to norm development—particularly the norms of self-disclosure so necessary for the successful small-group experience. The therapist has no more potent method to build behavioral norms than personal modeling.

Many of my own experiments in therapist self-disclosure originated as a response to the observation of therapy groups by students. Psychotherapy training programs rarely offer students an opportunity to observe individual psychotherapy sessions—therapists insist on the privacy and intimacy so integral to the individual therapy process. But almost every group training program provides for group observation either through a one-way mirror or video playback. The group therapists, of course, must obtain permission for observation, and group members will generally grant that permission but do so grudgingly. Characteristically, members resent the observers and often report feeling

like "guinea pigs." They question whether the primary allegiance of the therapist is to the group members or to the student observers, and they have great curiosity about the
observers' (and leader's) comments about them in the post-
group discussion.

To eliminate these disadvantages of group observation, I
asked the group members and the students to switch rooms
after each group meeting: the group members move into the
observation room, where they observe the students and me discussing the group. Group members, at the following meeting,
had such strong reactions to observing the post-group meeting
that I soon modified the format by inviting the members into
the conference room to observe the discussion and to respond
to the student observations. Soon the group members were giving feedback to students, not only about the content of the students' observations but about their process—for example, their
being too deferential to the leader, or more cautious, stiff, and
uptight than the therapy group.

I've used exactly the same model in daily groups on the
acute inpatient ward, where I divide the group meeting into
three parts: (1) a one-hour patient meeting; (2) a ten-minute
"fishbowl" session (the leaders and observers rehashing the
group while seated in an inner circle surrounded by the observing group members); and (3) a final ten-minute large circle in
which members react to the observers' comments. Debriefing
research indicates that most group members regard the final
twenty minutes as the most rewarding part of the meeting.

In another format for personal transparency, I routinely
write a detailed and impressionistic summary of outpatient
group meetings and mail it to members before the next meeting. This technique had its origins in the 1970s when I began
leading groups for alcoholic patients. All that time dynamic
group therapy for alcoholic patients had a bad reputation, and

most alcohol counselors had decided that it was best to leave alcoholic group treatment in the hands of AA. I decided to try once again but to employ an intensive here-and-now format and to shift the focus from the alcohol addiction to the underlying interpersonal problems that fueled the urge to drink. (All group members were required to participate in AA or some other program to control their drinking.)

The here-and-now focus galvanized the group. Meetings were electric and intensive. Unfortunately, far too intensive! Too much anxiety was aroused for members who, as many alcoholics do, had great difficulty binding and tolerating anxiety in any other manner but acting out. Members of the group soon began craving a drink after meetings and announcing, "If I ever have to sit through a meeting like the last one, I'll stop in the bar on the way home."

Since it seemed that the here-and-now meetings were on target and dealt with rich relevant issues for each group member, I sought to develop some method to help diminish the threat and anxiety of the sessions. I employed a series of techniques.

First, a here-and-now agenda written for each meeting on the blackboard containing such items as the following:

To enable John and Mary to continue examining their
    differences but to deal with each other in a less
    threatening and hurtful manner.
To help Paul request some group time to talk about
    himself.

Second, we used video playbacks of selected portions of the meetings.

Third, after each meeting I dictated and mailed to the members a weekly summary which was not only a narrative of the content of each session but also self-revealing. I described my experience in the group—my puzzlement, my pleasure with certain of my contributions, my chagrin at errors I had made, or issues I had overlooked, or members I felt I had neglected.

Of all these methods, the weekly summary was by far the most effective, and since then I have made a regular practice in my once-a-week groups to mail a detailed summary to the group members before the following meeting. (If I have a co-leader, we alternate responsibility for the summary.) The summary has many and diverse benefits—for example, it increases the continuity of the therapy work by plunging the group back into the themes of the previous meeting—but I cite it here because it provides a vehicle for therapist disclosure.

"Multiple therapy" is another disclosure-based teaching format I employed for several years, and in it two instructors and five students (psychiatric residents) interview a single patient for a series of six sessions. But rather than focus solely on the patient, we made a point to examine our own group process, including such issues as the students' style of asking questions, their relationship to one another and to the faculty leaders, the degree of competitiveness or empathy in the group. Obviously, given the economic crunch of health care today, multiple therapy has no economic future, but, as a teaching device, it demonstrated several effects of therapists' personal disclosure: it is good modeling for patients and encourages their own disclosure, it accelerates the therapy process, it demonstrates therapists' respect for the therapy process by their willingness to engage personally in it.

Recall the experiment in which I and a patient named Ginny exchanged our impressionistic summaries of each session. This format was also a challenging exercise in therapist transparency. The patient had so idealized me, had placed me on such an elevated pedestal, that a true meeting between us was not possible. Therefore, in my notes I deliberately attempted to reveal the very human feelings and experiences I had: my frustrations, my irritations, my insomnia, my vanity. This exercise, done early in my career, facilitated therapy and liberated me a good deal in subsequent therapeutic work.

A bold experiment in therapist transparency that has long intrigued me was conducted by Sándor Ferenczi (1873–1933), a Hungarian psychoanalyst who was a member of Freud's inner psychoanalytic circle and perhaps Freud's closest professional and personal confidant. Freud, more drawn to speculative questions about the application of psychoanalysis to the understanding of culture, was basically pessimistic about therapy and rarely tinkered with methods to improve therapy technique. Of all the analysts in the inner circle, it was Sándor Ferenczi who relentlessly and boldly sought out technical innovation.

He was never more bold than in his radical 1932 transparency experiment described in his *Clinical Diaries*, where he pushed therapist self-disclosure to the limit by engaging in "mutual analysis"—a format in which he and one of his patients (a female psychotherapist whom he had been analyzing for some time) alternated hours analyzing one another.

Ultimately Ferenczi grew discouraged and abandoned the experiment because of two major concerns: (1) *confidentiality*—a problem because true engagement in free association would require him to share any passing thoughts about his other patients and (2) *fees*—Ferenczi fretted about payment. Who should pay whom?

His patient did not share Ferenczi's discouragement. She felt the procedure had facilitated therapy and that Ferenczi was unwilling to continue because he feared having to acknowledge that he was in love with her. Ferenczi held a contrary opinion. "No, no, no," he opined; his real reason was that he was unwilling to express the fact that he hated her.

Ferenczi's negative reactions to his attempts at self-disclosure seem arbitrary and highly dated. My novel *Lying on the Couch* attempts to rerun his experiment in contemporary therapy. The protagonist, a psychiatrist, resolved to be totally transparent with a patient who, as it happened in this fictional tale, was committed to duplicity. One of my major intentions in the novel is to affirm that therapist authenticity will ultimately be redemptive even under the worst circumstances—that is, a clinical encounter with a scheming pseudo-patient.

CHAPTER 26

Three Kinds of Therapist Self-Disclosure

I t is counterproductive for the therapist to remain opaque and hidden from the patient. There is every reason to reveal oneself to the patient and no good reason for concealment. Yet whenever I begin to address therapists on this issue, I observe considerable discomfort, which stems in part from the imprecision of the term *self-disclosure*. Therapist self-disclosure is not a single entity but a cluster of behaviors, some of which invariably facilitate therapy and some of which are problematic and potentially counterproductive. Some clarity may be provided by delineating three realms of therapist disclosure: (1) the mechanism of therapy; (2) here-and-now feelings; and (3) the therapist's personal life. Let us examine each in turn.

CHAPTER 27

The Mechanism of Therapy— Be Transparent

The grand inquisitor in Dostoevsky's *Brothers Karamazov* proclaimed that men have always wanted "magic, mystery, and authority." Throughout history, healers have known this and cloaked their healing practice in a shroud of secrecy. Shamanistic training and practices have always been veiled in mystery, whereas Western physicians have, for centuries, used accoutrements designed to inspire awe and maximize a placebo effect: white coats, walls studded with prestigious diplomas, and prescriptions written in Latin.

I propose a diametrically opposed view of the healing process throughout this text. The establishment of an authentic relationship with patients, by its very nature, demands that we forgo the power of the triumvirate of magic, mystery, and authority. Psychotherapy is intrinsically so robust that it gains a great deal by full disclosure of the process and rationale of treatment. A persuasive body of psychotherapy research demonstrates that the therapist should carefully prepare new patients by informing them about psychotherapy—its basic assumptions, rationale, and what each client can do to maximize his or her own progress.

Patients are already burdened with the primary anxiety that brings them to therapy and it makes little sense to plunge them into a process that may create secondary anxiety—anxiety from exposure to an ambiguous social situation without guidelines for proper behavior or participation. Therefore it is wise to prepare patients systematically for the process of psychotherapy.

Preparation of new patients is particularly effective in group therapy because the interactional group situation is so intrinsically alien and frightening. New group members, especially those without previous group experience, are often made anxious by the power of the small group—the group pressure, the degree of intimacy, the overall intensity. The provision of anxiety-relieving structure and the clarification of procedural guidelines are absolutely essential in group therapy.

Preparation for individual psychotherapy is also essential. Though individuals are likely to have had experience with intense relationships, it is highly unlikely that they have been in a relationship requiring them to trust fully, to reveal all, to hold nothing back, to examine all nuances of their feelings to another, and to receive nonjudgmental acceptance. In initial interviews I cover important ground rules, including confidentiality, the necessity for full disclosure, the importance of dreams, the need for patience. Because the here-and-now focus may seem unusual to patients I present its rationale. If a new patient has described relationship difficulties (and that means just about every patient), I might say, for example:

> "It's clear that one of the areas we need to address is your relationship with others. It is difficult for me to know the precise nature of your difficulties in relationships because I, of course, know the other persons in

your life only through your own eyes. Sometimes your descriptions may be unintentionally biased, and I've found that I can be more helpful to you by focusing on the one relationship where I have the most accurate information—the relationship between you and me. It is for this reason I shall often ask you to examine what is happening between the two of us."

In short I suggest total disclosure about the mechanism of therapy.

CHAPTER 28

Revealing Here-and-Now Feelings—
Use Discretion

To engage in a genuine relationship with one's patient, it is essential to *disclose your feelings toward the patient in the immediate present.* But here-and-now disclosure should not be indiscriminate; transparency should not be pursued for its own sake. All comments must pass one test: Is this disclosure in the best interests of the patient? Over and again in this text I shall emphasize that your most valuable source of data is your own feelings. If during an hour you feel that the patient is distant, shy, flirtatious, scornful, fearful, challenging, childlike, or exhibiting any of a myriad of behaviors one person can with another, then that is data, valuable data, and you must seek a way to turn that information to therapeutic advantage, as shown in examples of my revealing that I felt shut out by a patient, or closer and more involved, or irritated at repetitive apologies for moving a Kleenex box.

Clinical illustration. A patient customarily described problematic incidents in his life but rarely gave me a follow-up. I often felt shut out and curious. I wondered what happened, for example, when he confronted his boss for a raise? What was his friend's reaction when he refused to give him the loan he requested? Did he follow through with his plan of asking his ex-girlfriend's roommate for a date? Perhaps some of my curiosity was voyeuristic, emanating from my desire to know the ends of stories. But I felt also my reactions contained important information about the patient. Did he never put himself in my position? Did he not think I had any curiosity about his life? Perhaps he felt he didn't matter to me. Perhaps he thought of me as a machine without any of my own curiosity and desires.

Ultimately I discussed all of these feelings (and conjectures), and my disclosure led him into revealing his preference that I not be a real person lest he discover my shortcomings and consequently lose confidence in me.

Clinical illustration. A patient experienced a sense of pervasive illegitimacy and shame in all his personal and business transactions. In the here-and-now of our therapy hours his free-floating guilt often emerged as he castigated himself for his inauthentic behavior in our relationship. He hated the way he tried to impress me with his cleverness and his intelligence. For example, he loved languages and, though English was his second language, he reveled in mastering its nuances and confessed that he had often searched the dictionary before sessions for esoteric words to use in our discussion. I felt dismayed at his self-castigation. For a moment I could experience the force of his guilt and self-criticism, since I was a full accomplice: I had always taken great delight in his wordplay and, without doubt, had encouraged his behavior. I shared that and then treated us both by exclaiming, "But I'm not buying into this. After all, where's the crime? We're working well together and what is the harm in our enjoying our shared intellectual play?"

A gifted therapist (Peter Lomas) describes the following interaction with a patient who began the session in his characteristic manner by speaking in a withdrawn and hopeless manner about his loneliness.

> THERAPIST: "Don't you think that I, too, might be lonely? Here I am sitting with you in this room and you are withdrawn from me. Don't you recognize that I don't want this, that I want to get to know you better?"
>
> PATIENT: "No, how could you? I can't believe it. You are self-sufficient. You don't want me."
>
> THERAPIST: "What makes you think I'm self-sufficient? Why should I be different from you? I need people like you do. And I need you to stop keeping away from me."
>
> PATIENT: "What could I give you? I can't imagine it. I feel so much a nothing. I never do anything in my life."
>
> THERAPIST: "But in any case one doesn't like people just because of their achievements but for what they are. Don't you?"
>
> PATIENT: "Yes, that's true for me."
>
> THERAPIST: "So why don't you believe that others might like you for what you are?"

The therapist reported that this interaction dramatically decreased the gulf between himself and the patient. The patient ended the hour saying, "It's a hard world," but his statement was delivered not in the sense of "poor unhappy me," but in the sense of "It's a hard world for you and me, isn't it, for you and me and all others who live in it?"

CHAPTER 29

Revealing the Therapist's Personal Life—Use Caution

Disclosure in the first two realms—the mechanism of therapy and the here-and-now (properly framed)— seems straightforward and nonproblematic. But around the third type of disclosure, the personal life of the therapist, there swirls considerable controversy.

If therapist disclosure were to be graded on a continuum, I am certain that I would be placed on the high end. Yet I have never had the experience of disclosing too much. On the contrary, I have always facilitated therapy when I have shared some facet of myself.

Many years ago my mother died, and I flew to Washington for her funeral and to spend time with my sister. I was leading an outpatient group at the time, and my co-therapist, a young psychiatric resident, was uncertain what to do and simply informed the group that I would be absent because of a death in my family. The group meetings were being videotaped for research and teaching purposes, and upon my return a week later I viewed the tape of the meeting—a productive, highly energized session.

What to do in the next meeting? Since I had no doubt that concealment of my mother's death would be deleterious to the group process, I decided to be entirely transparent and give the group everything they requested. It is axiomatic that if a group actively avoids some major issue, then no other issue will be addressed effectively.

I opened the meeting by informing them of my mother's death and responded to all inquiries. Some wanted to know details of the death and funeral, others asked about how I was handling it, others inquired about my relationship to my mother and sister. I answered all with great candor and told them, for example, of my fractious relationship with my mother and how I had chosen to live in California partly in order to put three thousand miles between my mother and me. She had been a dragon in many ways, I told them, but she had lost her fangs as she had aged and in the last several years our relationship had grown much closer and I had been a dutiful son. Finally the group asked whether there was anything they could do for me in the meeting. I responded that I didn't believe so because I had been dealing nonstop with my mother's death by talking intensively with friends and family. Finally, I said that I believed that I now had the energy to work effectively in the group, whereupon the group turned back to group business and had an extremely productive meeting.

For years afterward, I used the videotape of this meeting to teach group process. I feel certain that my disclosure not only removed a potential roadblock to the group but that my modeling self-disclosure was a liberating event for it.

Another example, which I described in a story, "Seven Advanced Lessons in the Therapy of Grief" (*Momma and the Meaning of Life*), involves a similar incident. Shortly before I was to meet with a bereaved patient, I received a call informing me of my brother-in-law's death. Since my patient was a surgeon in crisis (over the death of both her husband and her father), and I had time before leaving for the airport, I decided to keep my appointment with her, and opened the hour by informing her of what had happened and telling her that I had nonetheless decided to keep the appointment with her.

She exploded with great fury and accused me of attempting to compare my grief with hers. "And let me tell you," she added, "if I can show up in the operating room for my patients, then you sure as hell can show up to see me." The incident proved very instrumental for therapy—my revelation enabled her to reveal her grief rage, which opened a new fertile period in our work.

Long ago a colleague worked with a patient whose child had died of cancer. The long course of therapy had been helpful but not entirely successful. My colleague, who had also lost a young child twenty years earlier, chose not to share that information with his patient. Many years later the patient contacted him again and they resumed therapy. The therapist, who had continued to be haunted by his own loss and had spent years writing a long article on his child's death, decided to share the writing with the patient. This disclosure, which was novel for him, proved vastly instrumental in accelerating the therapy work.

If patients want to know whether I am married, have children, liked a certain movie, read a certain book, or felt awkward at our meeting at some social event, I always answer them directly. Why not? What's the big deal? How can one have a genuine encounter with another person while remaining so opaque?

Return, one final time, to the patient who was critical of me for using an upscale restaurant as a landmark for directions to my office while failing to mention the neighboring fast-food taco stand. I chose to respond candidly, "Well, Bob, you're right! Instead of saying turn right at Fresca, I could have said turn right when you reach the taco stand. And why did I make the choice I did? I'm sure it's because I'd rather associate myself with the more refined restaurant. I'd feel uncomfortable saying, 'Turn at the taco stand.'" Again, what's the risk? I'm only acknowledging something he obviously knew. And only when we got my admission out of the way could we turn to the important business of exploring his desire to embarrass me.

Thus, by no means does therapist self-disclosure replace the exploration of the process of the patient's personal inquiries. Do both! Some therapists make a point of responding to questions with: "I'll be glad to answer that, but first I'd like to know as much as possible about the asking of that question." Sometimes I use that approach, but I've rarely found particular advantage in insisting on any particular order ("You go first and then I'll respond"). If it is a new patient I often choose simply to model disclosure and to store the incident in my mind to return to later.

If it is unusual for the patient to ask you questions, then consider their act of questioning as grist for the mill and make certain you return to it. Timing must be considered. Often the therapist may choose to wait until the interaction is over, perhaps even until the next session, then remark to this effect: "It seems to me that something unusual happened last week: you asked me some personal questions. Can we revisit that? What was the exchange like for you? What enabled you to approach me in a different way? How did you feel about my response?"

CHAPTER 30

Revealing Your Personal Life—Caveats

One of the deepest fears therapists have about personal disclosure is that there will be no end to it, that once they open the door, the patient will demand more and more until they are being grilled about their deepest and most embarrassing secrets. This is a groundless fear. In my experience the overwhelming majority of patients accept what I offer, do not press for more or for uncomfortable disclosure, then go about the business of therapy, as the therapy group did upon learning of my mother's death.

However, there are caveats: Keep in mind that, though the patients have confidentiality, therapists do not. Nor can one request it of patients, who may in the future consult another therapist and must feel unencumbered in what they may discuss. If there is certain information that you strongly do not wish to become public, *do not share it in therapy.* Many therapists are even more cautious and take care not to share any personal material that, out of context, might be misconstrued and prove embarrassing.

But do not permit this concern to restrict your work and make you so overcautious and self-protective that you lose your effectiveness. You cannot protect yourself from patients' presenting you in distorted fashion to their next therapist. Keep this in mind the next time you hear patients describe the outrageous behavior of previous therapists. Don't automatically leap to the conclusion that the previous therapist was foolish or malfeasant. It is best to listen, empathize, and wait. Very often the patient will eventually provide the context of the therapist's act, which often throws it into a very different light.

I once referred a wife of a patient to a colleague, a close friend. But a couple of months later, my patient asked me for another referral because my colleague had acted badly: he had persisted in smelling my patient's wife and commenting upon her odor. Smelling patients? It sounded so bizarre that I felt concerned about my friend and as gently as possible inquired about the incident. He informed me that there had indeed been an odor problem with his patient: she customarily wore perfume that, though pleasing, was so powerful and pervasive that some of his other patients had complained and insisted on being seen some other day or in another office!

There are times when, in order to save the therapy, one is forced into tough choices. A colleague once told me of an incident in which a long-term patient came into a session highly distressed because a friend of hers had claimed to have had an affair with the therapist. How should the therapist respond? My colleague, who was committed to honesty, bit the bullet and told his patient that he had indeed had a weekend "convention affair" with this woman more than twenty years ago and that they had had no contact since. His disclosure had a considerable impact on her and galvanized subsequent therapy. He and his patient plunged into important, previously undiscussed issues such as her hatred of his other patients, whom she saw as competitors for his attention, and her lifelong view of herself as being unchosen, unfeminine, and unattractive.

Another example: A supervisee of mine, who was gay but had not come out, reported a vexing problem that arose in the first month of therapy. One of his gay patients who had seen him working out in a gym largely used by gay men confronted him directly about his sexual orientation. My student, highly uncomfortable, avoided the question by focusing upon the issue of why the patient was asking. Not surprisingly, the patient canceled his next session and never returned to therapy. Big, unconcealable secrets are inimical to the therapeutic process. The accomplished gay therapists I know are open about their sexual orientation with their gay clientele and are willing to be open with their straight clients if it seems important to the therapy.

CHAPTER 31

Therapist Transparency
and Universality

A key therapeutic factor in group therapy is universality. Many patients begin therapy feeling unique in their wretchedness; they believe they alone have thoughts and fantasies that are awful, forbidden, tabooed, sadistic, selfish, and sexually perverse. The self-disclosure of similar thoughts by other group members is wonderfully comforting and provides a "welcome to the human race" experience.

In individual therapy our patients disclose many feelings that we therapists have also experienced, and there is a place and a time in therapy for sharing these. If, for example, a patient expresses guilt over the fact that whenever she visits an aged parent she feels crawly with impatience after a couple hours, I may share that my personal limit for a sitting visit with my mother was about three hours. Or, if a patient is discouraged about feeling no better after twenty hours of therapy, I do not hesitate referring to that amount as a "drop in the bucket," considering my own hundreds of hours of treatment over several courses of therapy. Or if patients are bewildered by the intensity of transference, I tell them of my similar feelings when I was in therapy.

CHAPTER 32

Patients Will Resist
Your Disclosure

My earlier comment that the therapist's self-disclosure does not whet patients' appetites and cause them to escalate their demands for further disclosure is, in fact, an understatement. Very often the opposite takes place—patients make it clear they are opposed to learning much more about the personal life of the therapist.

Those who desire magic, mystery, and authority are loath to look beneath the trappings of the therapist. They are much comforted by the thought that there is a wise and omniscient figure to help them. More than one of my patients have invoked the metaphor of the Wizard of Oz to describe their preference for the happy belief that the therapist knows the way home—a clear, sure path out of pain. By no means do they want to look behind the curtain and see a lost and confused faux-wizard. One patient, who vacillated between "wizarding" and humanizing me, described the Oz dilemma in this poem entitled "Dorothy Surrenders":

My flight crash-landed on the Kansas plain
I woke to home-truths slashed in black and white.
Felt slippers, a life cutting along the grain,
And empty crystal. I tried. But neon nights
I'd searched for emeralds inside green glass,
For wizards behind straw men, I'd see
That horse of many colors gallop past—
And I grew old, he raced too fast for me.
The raging winds I've flown within have scraped
Me bare. Now on my knees I'd make the choice
To leave the witch her broom, replace the drape,
Refuse to see the man behind the voice
Forever following that magic road
That leads me to a place no place like home.

Patients want the therapist to be omniscient, infinitely dependable, and imperishable. Some of my female patients who have had many encounters with undependable men fear my (and all male) frailty. Others fear that I will wind up becoming the patient. One patient, whose course of therapy I described in depth in *Momma and the Meaning of Life*, avoided looking at me or asking me anything personal, even, for example, when I appeared at a session on crutches after knee surgery. When I inquired she explained:

> "I don't want you to have a narrative to your life."
> "A narrative?" I asked. "What do you mean?"
> "I want to keep you outside time. A narrative has a beginning, a middle, and an end—especially an end."

She had suffered the death of several important men in her life—her husband, brother, father, godson—and was terrified at the prospect of another loss. I responded that I could not help her without our having a human encounter; I needed for her to regard me as a real person and prodded her into asking me questions about my life and my health. After leaving my office that day, she had an obsessive thought: *The next funeral I attend will be Irv's.*

CHAPTER 33

Avoid the Crooked Cure

What is the crooked cure? It is a term used in the early days of psychoanalysis to refer to a transference cure—a sudden radical improvement in the patient based on magic, emanating from an illusory view of the power of the therapist.

A forty-five-year-old single, isolated woman often left my office glowing with a deep sense of well-being that persisted for days after each session. At first I could only welcome her relief from months of black despair. And welcome also her heady comments about me: the many insights I offered her, my extraordinary prescience. But soon, as she described how between therapy hours she draped me around her like a magic protective cloak, how she filled herself with courage and peace merely by hearing my taped voice on my answering machine, I grew more and more uncomfortable with shaman powers.

Why? For one thing, I knew I was encouraging regression by ignoring that her improvement was built on shifting sand, and that as soon as I disappeared from her life, her improvement would evaporate. I also grew uncomfortable with the unreal and inauthentic nature of our relationship. The more her symptoms receded, the broader and deeper the fissure between us grew.

Eventually I confronted the issue and explained that much of her experience in our relationship was of her own construction—that is, I was not privy to it. I told her everything: that I was not really draped around her shoulders like a magic cloak, that I did not share in many of the epiphanies she had experienced in our hours, that I liked being so important to her but at the same time felt fraudulent. All the magical help she had obtained from me? Well, it was she, not I, who was the magician, she who had really given this help to herself.

My comments, she told me later, felt powerful, cruel, and disorienting. However, she had by that time changed enough to integrate the idea that her improvement came not from my power but from sources within herself. Moreover, she ultimately came to an understanding that my comments were not a rejection but, on the contrary, an invitation to relate to me more closely and more honestly.

Perhaps there are times when we must provide "magic, mystery, and authority"—times of great crisis or times when our chief priority is to ease the patient into therapy. But if we must flirt with the role of wizard I advise that we keep the flirtation brief and set about helping the patient quickly make the transition into a more genuine therapeutic relationship.

A patient who had idealized me early in therapy dreamed two dreams one night: In the first, a tornado approached and I led her and others up a fire escape that ultimately dead-ended against a brick wall. In the second dream she and I were taking an examination and neither of us knew the answers. I welcomed these dreams because they informed the patient of my limits, my humanness, my having to grapple with the same fundamental problems of life that she did.

CHAPTER 34

On Taking Patients Further
Than You Have Gone

Often when I encounter a patient struggling with some of the same neurotic issues that have hounded me throughout life, I question whether I can take my patient further than I myself have come.

There are two opposing points of view: An older, traditional analytic view, less in evidence today, holds that only the thoroughly analyzed therapist can escort patients to a complete resolution of neurotic problems, whereas the blind spots of clinicians with unresolved neurotic issues limit the amount of help they are able to provide.

One of Nietzsche's aphorisms expresses an opposing view: "Some cannot loosen their own chains yet can nonetheless redeem their friends." Karen Horney's view of the self-actualizing drive (undoubtedly emerging from Nietzsche's work) is relevant: if the therapist removes obstacles, patients will naturally mature and realize their potential, even attaining a level of integration beyond that of the facilitating therapist. I find this view far more consonant with my experience in working with patients. Indeed I have often had patients whose change and whose courage have left me gaping in admiration.

There exists in the world of letters considerable analogous data. Some of the most important *lebens-philosophers* (philosophers dealing with problems inherent in existence) were singularly tormented individuals. For starters, consider Nietzsche and Schopenhauer (extraordinarily isolated, anguished souls), Sartre (alcohol and drug abuser, interpersonally exploitative and insensitive), and Heidegger (who wrote so profoundly on authenticity yet supported the Nazi cause and betrayed his own colleagues, including Husserl, his teacher).

The same point may be made for many of the early psychologists whose substantial contributions have been so useful to so many: Jung, no paragon of interpersonal skills, was sexually exploitative of patients, as were many of the members of Freud's inner circle—for example, Ernest Jones, Otto Rank, and Sándor Ferenczi. Consider, too, the astounding amount of discord characteristic of all the major psychoanalytic institutes, whose members, despite their expertise in assisting others, have at the same time characteristically displayed so much immaturity, mutual acrimony, and disrespect that schism after schism has occurred, with new—and often feuding—institutes spinning wildly off from mother institutes.

CHAPTER 35

On Being Helped by Your Patient

In a play fragment, *Emergency,* the psychoanalyst Helmut Kaiser tells the story of a wife who visits a therapist and pleads with him to help her husband, a psychiatrist who is deeply depressed and likely to kill himself. The therapist responds that of course he would be glad to help and suggests that her husband call for an appointment. The woman responds that therein lies the problem: Her husband denies his depression and rejects all suggestions to obtain help. The therapist is baffled. He tells the woman that he cannot imagine how he can be of help to someone unwilling to consult him.

The woman replies that she has a plan. She urges the psychiatrist to consult her husband, while pretending to be a patient, and gradually, as they continue to meet, find a way to help him.

These and other tales as well as my clinical experience informed the plot of my novel *When Nietzsche Wept,* in which Friedrich Nietzsche and Josef Breuer served simultaneously (and surreptitiously) as each other's therapist and patient.

I believe it is commonplace for therapists to be helped by

their patients. Jung often spoke of the increased efficacy of the wounded healer. He even claimed that therapy worked best when the patient brought the perfect salve for the therapist's wound and that if the therapist doesn't change, then the patient doesn't, either. Perhaps wounded healers are effective because they are more able to empathize with the wounds of the patient; perhaps it is because they participate more deeply and personally in the healing process.

I know that I have, countless times, begun a therapy hour in a state of personal disquiet and ended the hour feeling considerably better without commenting explicitly on my inner state. I think help has come to me in many forms. Sometimes it is the result of sheerly being effective in my work, of feeling better about myself through using my skills and expertise to help another. Sometimes it ensues from being drawn out of myself and into contact with another. Intimate interaction is always salutary.

I have especially encountered this phenomenon in my group-therapy practice. Many times I have started a therapy-group session feeling troubled about some personal issue and finished the meeting feeling considerably relieved. The intimate healing ambiance of a good therapy group is almost tangible, and good things occur when one enters into its aura. Scott Rutan, an eminent group therapist, once compared the therapy group to a bridge built during a battle. Though there may be some casualties sustained during the stage of building (i.e., group-therapy dropouts), the bridge, once in place, can transport a great many people to a better place.

These are by-products of healers' doing their job, times when the healer is surreptitiously taking in some of that good stuff of therapy. Sometimes the healer's therapy is more explicit and transparent. Even though the patient is not there to treat the therapist, times may arise when the therapist is burdened with sorrows that are difficult to conceal. Bereavement is perhaps the most common sorrow, and many a patient has sought to bolster the spirits of the bereaved therapist, as in the example I cited earlier of my therapy group's response to my mother's death. I also remember each of my individual patients at that time reaching out to me in a human fashion—and not just to help tune me up so that I could more efficiently attend to their therapy.

After the publication of *Love's Executioner* I received a critical review in *The New York Times Book Review* and a very positive review later in the week in the daily *New York Times*. Several of my patients left messages for me or began their next session by asking me if I had seen the positive review and commiserating with me about the negative one. On another occasion, following a particularly mean-spirited newspaper interview, one patient reminded me that the newspaper would be used to wrap fish the following day.

Harry Stack Sullivan, an influential American psychiatric theorist, is reputed to have once described psychotherapy as a discussion of personal issues between two people, one of them more anxious than the other. And if the therapist develops more anxiety than the patient, *he* becomes the patient and the patient becomes the therapist. Furthermore, the patient's self-esteem is radically boosted by being of help to the therapist. I have had several opportunities to minister to important figures in my life. In one case I was able to offer consolation to a despairing mentor and was then called upon to treat his son. In another, I often advised and comforted an elderly former therapist, saw him through a lengthy illness, and was privileged to be at his side at the moment of his death. Despite revealing the frailty of my elders, these experiences served to enrich and strengthen me.

CHAPTER 36

Encourage Patient Self-Disclosure

elf-disclosure is an absolutely essential ingredient in psychotherapy. No patient profits from therapy without self-revelation. It is one of those automatic occurrences in therapy of which we take note only in its absence. So much of what we do in therapy—providing a safe environment, establishing trust, exploring fantasies and dreams—serves the purpose of encouraging self-revelation.

When a patient takes the plunge, breaks significant new ground, and reveals something new, something particularly difficult to discuss—something potentially embarrassing, shameful, or incriminating—then I make a point of focusing on the *process* of the comment as well as its *content*. (Keep in mind that *process* refers to the nature of the relationship between the people in the interaction.) In other words, at some point, often after a full discussion of the content, I make sure to turn my attention to the patient's act of disclosure. First I take care to treat such a disclosure tenderly and comment on how I feel about the patient's willingness to trust me. I then turn my attention to the decision to share this material with me at this time.

The construct of "vertical disclosure versus horizontal disclosure" may help to clarify this point. *Vertical disclosure* refers to in-depth disclosure about the content of the disclosure. If the disclosure has to do, let us say, with sexual stimulation from cross-dressing, then the therapist might encourage vertical disclosure by inquiring about the historical development of the cross-dressing or the particular details and circumstances of the practice—that is, what the patient wears, what fantasies are used, whether it is solitary or shared, and so on.

Horizontal disclosure, on the other hand, is *disclosure about the act of disclosure*. To facilitate horizontal disclosure we ask such questions as "What made it possible to discuss this today? How hard was it for you? Had you been wanting to share this in earlier sessions? What stopped you? I imagine that since there is just you and me here it must have something to do with how you anticipate I would respond to you. [Patients usually agree with this self-evident truth.] How did you anticipate I'd respond? What response have you seen from me today? Are there any questions about my response you'd like to ask me?"

In group therapy the process of self-disclosure enters into particularly sharp focus because differences between the group members are so evident. With considerable consensus, group members can rank their fellow members according to transparency. Ultimately groups become impatient with withholding members, and the unwillingness to disclose becomes a major focus in the group.

Often members respond impatiently to long-delayed disclosures. "*Now* you tell us about the affair you've been having the last three years," they say. "But what about that wild-goose chase you took us on the last six months? Look at the time we wasted—all those meetings in which we assumed your marriage was falling apart solely because of your wife's coldness and disinterest in you. This process requires active intervention by the therapist because patients should not be punished for self-revelation, no matter how delayed. It is the same for individual therapy. Anytime you feel like saying, "Dammit, all these wasted hours, why didn't you tell me this before," that is just the time to bite your tongue and shift the focus onto the fact that the patient *did* finally develop the trust to reveal this information.

CHAPTER 37

Feedback in Psychotherapy

The Johari window, a venerable personality paradigm used in teaching group leaders and group members about self-disclosure and feedback, has much to offer in individual therapy as well. Its odd name is a conflation (Joe + Harry) of the two individuals who first described it—Joe Luft and Harry Ingram. Note the four quadrants: public, blind, secret, unconscious.

	Known to Self	Unknown to Self
Known to Others	1. public	2. blind
Unknown to Others	3. secret	4. unconscious

Quadrant 1 (*known to myself and to others*) is the public self.

Quadrant 2 (*unknown to self and known by others*) is the blind self.

Quadrant 3 (*known to self and unknown to others*) is the secret self.

Quadrant 4 (*unknown to self and to others*) is the unconscious self.

The quadrants vary in size between individuals: Some cells are large in some individuals, shrunken in others. In therapy we attempt to change the size of the four cells. We try to help the public cell grow larger at the expense of the other three and the secret self to shrink, as patients, through the process of self-disclosure, share more of themselves—at first to the therapist and then judiciously to other appropriate figures in their lives. And, of course, we hope to diminish the size of the unconscious self by helping patients explore and become acquainted with deeper layers of themselves.

But it is cell 2, the *blind self*, that we particularly target—both in individual and group therapy. A goal of therapy is to increase reality testing and to help individuals see themselves as others see them. It is through the agency of feedback that the *blind self* cell grows appreciably smaller.

In group therapy, feedback for the most part is from member to member. In group sessions members interact a great deal with others, and considerable data is generated about interpersonal patterns. If the group is conducted properly, members receive much feedback from the other group members about how they are perceived by them. But feedback is a delicate tool and members soon learn that it is most useful if:

1. It stems from here-and-now observations.
2. It follows the generating event as closely as possible.
3. It focuses on the specific observations and feelings generated in the listener rather than guesses or interpretations about the speaker's motivation.
4. The recipient checks out the feedback with other members to obtain consensual validation.

In the two-person system of individual therapy, feedback is less variegated and voluminous but is nonetheless an instrumental part of the therapy process. It is through feedback that patients become better witnesses to their own behavior and learn to appreciate the impact of their behavior upon the feelings of others.

CHAPTER 38

Provide Feedback Effectively
and Gently

If you have some clear here-and-now impressions that seem germane to the central issues of your patient, you must develop modes of delivering these observations in a manner the patient can accept.

There are steps I find useful early in the course of therapy. First, I enlist the patient as an ally and request his permission to offer my here-and-now observations. Then I make it clear that these observations are highly relevant to the patient's reasons for being in therapy. For example, in one of the first sessions I might say:

> "Perhaps I can help you understand what goes wrong with relationships in your life by examining our relationship as it is occurring. Even though our relationship is not the same as a friendship, there is, nonetheless, much overlap, particularly the intimate nature of our discussion. If I can make observations about you that might

throw light on what happens between you and others, I'd
like to point them out. Is that okay?"

It is hardly possible for the patient to reject this offer, and
once we have nailed down this contract, I feel bolder and less
intrusive when giving feedback. As a general rule, such an
agreement is a good idea, and I may remind the patient of our
contract if awkwardness should arise about feedback.

Consider, for example, these three patients:
Ted who for months speaks in a soft voice and refuses to
      meet my glance.
Bob, an efficient, high-powered CEO, who comes to each
      session with a written agenda, takes notes during the
      session, and asks me to repeat many of my statements so
      as not to miss a word.
Sam, who rambles and continually spins long, tangential,
      pointless tales.

Each of these three patients reported great difficulty in
forming intimate relationships, and in each instance their here-
and-now behavior was obviously relevant to their relationship
problems. The task, in each instance, was to find a suitable
method of sharing my impressions.

"Ted, I'm very much aware of the fact that you never
meet my glance. I don't, of course, know *why* you look
away, but I am aware that it prompts me to speak to you
very gently, almost as though you are fragile and that
sense of your fragility prompts me to weigh carefully
everything I say to you. I believe this caution prevents me
from being spontaneous and feeling close to you. Do my

comments surprise you? Perhaps you've heard this before?"

"Bob, let me share a couple of feelings. Your note-taking and the agendas you bring to sessions signify to me how hard you're working to make good use of this time. I appreciate your dedication and preparation but at the same time these activities have a definite impact on me. I'm aware of a highly businesslike, rather than a personal, atmosphere in our meetings, and also I often feel so closely scrutinized and evaluated that my spontaneity is stifled. I find that I am more cautious with you than I'd like to be. Is it possible you affect others in the same way?"

"Sam, let me interrupt you. You're into a long tale and I'm beginning to feel lost—I'm losing sight of its relevance to our work. Many of your stories are tremendously interesting. You're a very good storyteller and I get involved in your narratives but at the same time they operate as a barrier between us. The stories keep me away from you and they prevent a deeper encounter. Is this something that you've heard before from others?"

Note carefully the wording in these responses. In each I stick to my observations of the behavior I see and how that behavior makes me feel. I take care to avoid guesses about what the patient is attempting to do—that is, I do not comment that the patient is attempting to avoid me by not looking at me, or control me by the written agendas, or entertain me by the long stories. If I focus upon my own feelings, then I am far less likely to evoke defensiveness—after all, they are *my* feelings and cannot be challenged. In each instance I also introduce the idea that it is my wish to be closer to these patients and to know them better, that the behavior in question distances me and may distance others as well.

CHAPTER 39

Increase Receptiveness to Feedback by Using "Parts"

few other suggestions about feedback. Avoid giving generalized feedback; instead make it focused and explicit. Avoid simply responding affirmatively to general questions from patients about whether you like them. Instead, increase the usefulness of your response by reframing the question and discussing the aspects of the patient that draw you closer and those that push you away.

Using "parts" is often a helpful device to decrease defensiveness. Consider, for example, a patient who is almost always late in paying his bill. Whenever discussing it he is painfully embarrassed and offers many lame excuses. I've found formulations like the following useful:

> "Dave, I understand there may be realistic reasons for your not paying my bill on time. I do realize that you work hard in therapy, that you value me, and that you have found our work valuable. But I also think there is some

small resistant part of you that has some strong feelings about paying me. Please, I'd like to speak to that part."

Using "parts" is a useful concept to undermine denial and resistance in many phases of therapy and is often a gracious and gentle way to explore ambivalence. Furthermore, for patients who cannot tolerate ambivalence and tend to see life in black-and-white terms, it is an effective introduction to the notion of shades of gray.

For example, consider one of my gay patients who is reckless about unprotected sex and offers a number of rationalizations. My approach was, "John, I understand that you believe that in this situation your chance of getting HIV is only one in fifteen hundred. But I also know there is some particularly reckless or careless part of you. I want to meet and to converse with that part—that fifteen hundredth part of you."

Or to a despondent or suicidal patient: "I understand that you feel deeply discouraged, that at times you feel like giving up, that right now you even feel like taking your life. But you are nonetheless here today. Some part of you has brought the rest of you into my office. Now, please, I want to talk to that part of you—the part that wants to live."

CHAPTER 40

Feedback:
Strike When the Iron Is Cold

A new patient, Bonny, enters my office. She is forty, attractive, and has a face that is angelic and gleams as though it has just been freshly scrubbed. Though she is popular and has many friends, she tells me she is always left behind. Men are glad to go to bed with her but invariably choose to pass out of her life in a few weeks. "Why?" she asks. "Why does no one take me seriously?"

In my office she is always bubbly and enthusiastic and reminds me of a lively tour guide or an adorable tail-wagging puppy. She seems a young kid—clean, fun-loving, uncomplicated, but most unreal and uninteresting. It is not difficult to understand why others fail to take her seriously.

I am certain my observations are important and that I should make use of them in therapy. But how? How can I avoid hurting her and causing her to close down and become defensive? One principle that has proved useful to me time and again is to *strike when the iron is cold*—that is, give her the feedback about this behavior when she is behaving differently.

For example, one day she wept bitterly in my office as she spoke about attending the wedding of her younger sister. Life was passing her by; her friends were all marrying while she did nothing but age. Quickly composing herself, she beamed a huge smile and apologized for "being a baby" and letting herself get so down in my office. I took the opportunity to tell her that not only were apologies unnecessary but, on the contrary, it was particularly important for her to share with me her times of despair.

"I feel," I said, "much closer to you today. You seem much more real. It's as though I really know you now—better than ever before."

Silence.

"Your thoughts, Bonny?"

"You mean, I've got to break down for you to feel you know me?"

"I can see how you'd think that. Let me explain. There are many times when you come into my office and I have the sense of you being sparkling and entertaining; yet somehow I feel far away from the real you. There is a certain effervescence you have at these times that is very charming but it also acts as a barrier, keeping us apart. Today it's different. Today I feel really connected to you—and my hunch is this is the type of connection you yearn for in your social relationships. Tell me, does my reaction feel bizarre? Or familiar? Anyone else ever said this to you? Is it possible that what I'm saying might have some relevance to what goes on with you in other relationships?"

Another related technique employs age states. Sometimes I experience a patient as being in one age state, sometimes another, and I try to find an acceptable way to share this with the patient, usually commenting upon it when I experience the patient in an age-appropriate state. Some patients find this concept particularly important and may monitor themselves frequently and speak about what age they feel during a given session.

CHAPTER 41

Talk About Death

The fear of death always percolates beneath the surface. It haunts us throughout life and we erect defenses— many based on denial—to help cope with the awareness of death. But we cannot keep it out of mind. It spills over into our fantasies and dreams. It bursts loose in every nightmare. When we were children we were preoccupied with death and one of our major developmental tasks has been to cope with the fear of obliteration.

Death is a visitor in every course of therapy. To ignore its presence gives the message that it is too terrible to discuss. Yet most therapists avoid direct discussion of death. Why? Some therapists avoid it because they don't know what to do with death. "What's the point?" they say. "Let's get back to the neurotic process, something we can do something about." Other therapists question the relevance of death to the therapy process and follow the counsel of the great Adolph Meyer, who advised not scratching where it doesn't itch. Still others decline to bring up a subject that inspires great anxiety in an already anxious patient (and in the therapist as well).

Yet there are several good reasons we should confront death in the course of therapy. First, keep in mind that therapy is a deep and comprehensive exploration into the course and meaning of one's life; given the centrality of death in our existence, given that life and death are interdependent, how can we possibly ignore it? From the beginning of written thought humans have realized that everything fades, that we fear the fading, and that we must find a way to live despite the fear and the fading. Psychotherapists cannot afford to ignore the many great thinkers who have concluded that learning to live well is to learn to die well.

CHAPTER 42

Death and Life Enhancement

Most mental health workers who tend to the dying have, during their training, been advised to read Tolstoy's story "The Death of Ivan Ilyich." Ivan Ilyich, a mean-spirited bureaucrat dying in agony, stumbles upon a stunning insight at the very end of his life: he realizes he is dying so badly because he has lived so badly. His insight begets great personal change, and in his last days Ivan Ilyich's life is flooded with a peace and meaningfulness that he had never achieved previously. Many other great works of literature contain a similar message. For example, in *War and Peace*, Pierre, the protagonist, is transformed after a last-second reprieve from a firing squad. Scrooge in *A Christmas Carol* does not suddenly become a new man because of Yuletide cheer; rather his transformation occurs when the spirit of the future permits him to witness his own death and the strangers squabbling over his possessions. The message in all these works is simple and profound: Though the physicality of death destroys us, the idea of death may save us.

In the years I worked with terminally ill patients, I saw a great many patients who, facing death, underwent significant and positive personal change. Patients felt they had grown wise; they re-prioritized their values and began to trivialize the trivia in their lives. It was as though cancer cured neurosis—phobias and crippling interpersonal concerns seemed to melt away.

I always had students observe my groups of cancer patients. Ordinarily, in a teaching institution, groups will permit student observation but do so grudgingly and often with some smoldering resentment. But not my groups of patients terminally ill with cancer! On the contrary, they welcomed the opportunity to share what they had learned. "But what a pity," I heard so many patients lament, "that we had to wait until now, until our bodies are riddled with cancer, to learn how to live."

Heidegger spoke of two modes of existence: the everyday mode and the ontological mode. In the everyday mode we are consumed with and distracted by material surroundings—we are filled with wonderment about *how things are* in the world. In the ontological mode we are focused on being per se—that is, we are filled with wonderment *that things are* in the world. When we exist in the ontological mode—the realm beyond everyday concerns—we are in a state of particular readiness for personal change.

But how do we shift from the everyday mode to the ontological mode? Philosophers often speak of "boundary experiences"—urgent experiences that jolt us out of "everydayness" and rivet our attention upon "being" itself. The most powerful boundary experience is a confrontation with one's own death. But what about boundary experiences in everyday clinical practice? How does the therapist obtain the leverage for change available in the ontological mode in patients not facing imminent death?

Every course of therapy is studded with experiences that, though less dramatic, may still effectively alter perspective.

Bereavement, dealing with the death of the other, is a boundary experience whose power is too rarely harnessed in the therapeutic process. Too often in bereavement work we focus extensively and exclusively upon loss, upon unfinished business in the relationship, upon the task of detaching ourselves from the dead and entering again into the stream of life. Though all these steps are important, we must not neglect the fact that the death of the other also serves to confront each of us, in a stark and poignant manner, with our own death. Years ago in a study of bereavement, I found that many bereaved spouses went further than simply undergoing repair and returning to their pre-bereavement level of functioning: between a fourth and a third of the subjects achieved a new level of maturity and wisdom.

In addition to death and bereavement, there arise many other opportunities for death-related discourse during the course of every therapy. If such issues never emerge, I believe the patient is simply following the therapist's covert instructions. Death and mortality form the horizon for all discussions about aging, bodily changes, life stages, and many significant life markers, such as major anniversaries, departure of children for college, the empty-nest phenomenon, retirement, the birth of grandchildren. A class reunion can be a particularly potent catalyst. Every patient discusses, at one time or another, newspaper accounts of accidents, atrocities, obituaries. And then, too, there is death's unmistakable footprint in every nightmare.

CHAPTER 43

How to Talk About Death

I prefer to speak of death directly and matter-of-factly. Early in the course of therapy I make a point of obtaining a history of my patients' experiences with death and ask such questions as When did you first become aware of death? With whom did you discuss it? How did adults in your life respond to your questions? What deaths have you experienced? Funerals attended? Religious beliefs regarding death? How have your attitudes about death changed during your life? Strong fantasies and dreams about death?

I approach patients with severe death anxiety in the same direct manner. A calm, matter-of-fact dissection of the anxiety is often reassuring. Often it is useful to dissect the fear and calmly inquire about what precisely is terrifying about death. Answers to this question generally include fears of the dying process, concerns for survivors, concerns about the afterlife (which beg the question by transforming death into a nonterminal event), and concerns about obliteration.

Once therapists demonstrate their personal equanimity

when discussing death, their patients will raise the topic far more frequently. For example, Janice, a thirty-two-year-old mother of three, had had a hysterectomy two years before. Preoccupied with having more children, she was jealous of other young mothers, angry when she was invited to showers of friends, and broke entirely with her pregnant best friend because of deep and bitter envy.

Our initial sessions focused on her relentless desire for more children and its ramifications on so many spheres of her life. In the third session I asked her whether she knew what she would be thinking about if she weren't thinking about having babies.

"Let me show you," Janice said. She opened her purse, pulled out a tangerine, peeled it, offered me a segment (which I accepted), and ate the rest.

"Vitamin C," she said. "I eat four tangerines a day."

"And why is vitamin C so important?"

"Prevents me from dying. Dying—that's the answer to your question about what I'd be thinking about. I think of dying all the time."

Death had haunted Janice since she was thirteen, when her mother had died. Filled with anger toward her mother for becoming sick, she had refused to visit her in the hospital during the last weeks of her life. Shortly afterward, she panicked because she thought a coughing episode indicated lung cancer and could not be reassured by emergency room physicians. Because her mother had died of breast cancer, Janice attempted to retard the growth of breasts by binding her chest and sleeping on her stomach. Guilt for abandoning her mother marked her for life, and she believed that dedicating herself to children was an atonement for not having taken care of her mother, as well as a mode of ensuring that she would not die alone.

Keep in mind that concerns about death often masquerade in sexual garb. Sex is the great death-neutralizer, the absolute vital antithesis of death. Some patients who are exposed to the great threat of death suddenly become pervasively preoccupied with sexual thoughts. (There are TAT [Thematic Appreciation Tests] studies documenting increased sexual content in cancer patients.) The French term for orgasm, *la petite mort* ("little death"), signifies the orgasmic loss of the self, which eliminates the pain of separateness—the lonely "I" vanishing into the merged "we."

A patient with a malignant abdominal cancer once consulted me because she had become infatuated with her surgeon to the extent that sexual fantasies about him replaced her fears about death. When, for example, she was scheduled for an important MRI, at which he would be present, the decision of which clothes to wear so consumed her that she lost sight of the fact that her life hung in the balance.

Another patient, an "eternal puer," a mathematical wunderkind with great potential, had remained childlike and closely attached to his mother well into his adult years. Extraordinarily gifted at conceiving great ideas, at impromptu brainstorming, at quickly grasping the essentials of complex new fields of inquiry, he never could muster the resolve to complete a project, to build a career, family, or household. Death concerns were not conscious but entered into our discussions via a dream:

> "My mother and I are in a large room. It resembles a room from our old house, yet it has a beach for one of the walls. We walk onto the beach and my mother urges me to go into the water. I am reluctant, but I get her a small chair to sit on and wade in. The water is very dark and

soon, as I go in deeper, up to my shoulders, the waves turn to granite. I wake up gasping for air and soaked in sweat."

The image of the granite waves covering him, a powerful image of terror, death, and burial, helped us to understand his reluctance to leave childhood and mother and to enter fully into adulthood.

CHAPTER 44

Talk About Life Meaning

We humans appear to be meaning-seeking creatures who have had the misfortune of being thrown into a world devoid of intrinsic meaning. One of our major tasks is to invent a meaning sturdy enough to support a life and to perform the tricky maneuver of denying our personal authorship of this meaning. Thus we conclude instead that it was "out there" waiting for us. Our ongoing search for substantial meaning systems often throws us into crises of meaning.

More individuals seek therapy because of concerns about meaning in life than therapists often realize. Jung reported that one-third of his patients consulted him for that reason. The complaints take many different forms: for example, "My life has no coherence," "I have no passion for anything," "Why am I living? To what end?" "Surely life must have some deeper significance." "I feel so empty—watching TV every night makes me feel so pointless, so useless." "Even now at the age of fifty I still don't know what I want to do when I grow up."

I once had a dream (described in *Momma and the Meaning*

of Life) in which, while hovering near death in a hospital room, I suddenly found myself on an amusement park ride (the House of Horrors). As the cart was just about to enter the black maw of death, I suddenly caught sight of my dead mother in the watching crowd and called out to her, "Momma, Momma, how'd I do?"

The dream, and especially my call—"Momma, Momma, how'd I do?"—haunted me for a long time, not because of the dream's death imagery, but because of its dark implications about life meaning. Was it possible, I wondered, that I had been conducting my whole life with the primary goal of obtaining my mother's approval? Because I had a troubled relationship with my mother and did not value her approval when she was alive, the dream was that much more mordant.

The crisis of meaning depicted in the dream prompted me to explore my life in a different manner. In a story I wrote directly after the dream, I engaged in a conversation with my mother's ghost in order to heal the breach between us and to understand how our life meanings both intertwined and conflicted with one another.

Some experiential workshops use devices to encourage discourse about life meaning. Perhaps the most common is to ask participants what they might wish for their tombstone epitaph. Most such inquiries into life meaning lead to a discussion of such goals as altruism, hedonism, dedication to a cause, generativity, creativity, self-actualization. Many feel that meaning projects take on a deeper, more powerful significance if they are self-transcendent—that is, directed at something or someone outside themselves, such as the love of a cause, a person, a divine essence.

The precocious recent success of young high-tech millionaires often generates a life crisis that can be instructive about non-self-transcendent life-meaning systems. Many such individuals begin their careers with a clear vision—making it, earning a pile of money, living the good life, receiving the respect of colleagues, retiring early. And an unprecedented number of young people in their thirties did exactly that. But then the question arose: "What now? What about the rest of my life—the next forty years?"

Most of the young high-tech millionaires that I have seen continue doing much of the same: they start new companies, try to repeat their success. Why? They tell themselves they must prove it was no fluke, that they can do it alone, without a particular partner or mentor. They raise the bar. To feel that they and their family are secure, they no longer need one or two million in the bank—they need five, ten, even fifty million to feel secure. They realize the pointlessness and irrationality in earning more money when they already have more than they can possibly spend, but this does not stop them. They realize they are taking away time from their families, from things closer to the heart, but they just cannot give up playing the game. "The money is just lying out there," they tell me. "All I have to do is pick it up." They have to make deals. One real estate entrepreneur told me that he felt he would disappear if he stopped. Many fear boredom—even the faintest whiff of boredom sends them scurrying right back to the game. Schopenhauer said that willing itself is never fulfilled—as soon as one wish is satisfied, another appears. Though there may be some very brief respite, some fleeting period of satiation, it is immediately transformed into boredom. "Every human life," he said, "is tossed backward and forward between pain and boredom."

Unlike my approach to other existential ultimate concerns (death, isolation, freedom), I find that meaning in life is best approached obliquely. What we must do is to plunge into one of many possible meanings, particularly one with a self-transcendent basis. It is engagement that counts, and we therapists do most good by identifying and helping to remove the obstacles to engagement. The question of meaning in life is, as the Buddha taught, not edifying. One must immerse oneself into the river of life and let the question drift away.

CHAPTER 45

Freedom

Earlier I described four ultimate concerns, four fundamental facts of existence—death, isolation, meaninglessness, freedom—which, when confronted, evoke deep anxiety. The linkage between "freedom" and anxiety is not intuitively apparent because at first glance "freedom" seems to contain only straightforward positive connotations. After all, have we not throughout the course of Western civilization yearned and struggled for political freedom? Yet freedom has a darker side. Viewed from the perspective of self-creation, choice, will, and action, freedom is psychologically complex and permeated with anxiety.

We are, in the deepest sense, responsible for ourselves. We are, as Sartre put it, the authors of ourselves. Through the accretion of our choices, our actions, and our failures to act, we ultimately design ourselves. We cannot avoid this responsibility, this freedom. In Sartre's terms, "we are condemned to freedom."

Our freedom runs even deeper than our individual life design. Over two centuries ago Kant taught us that we are responsible for providing form and meaning not only to the internal but to the external world as well. We encounter the external world only as it is processed though our own neurological and psychological apparatus. Reality is not at all as we imagined in childhood—we do not enter into (and ultimately leave) a well-structured world. Instead, we play the central role in constituting that world—and we constitute it as though it appears to have an independent existence.

And the relevance of freedom's dark side to anxiety and to clinical work? One answer can be found by looking down. If we are primal world constituters, then where is the solid ground beneath us? What is beneath us? Nothingness, *Das Nichts,* as the German existential philosophers put it. The chasm, the abyss of freedom. And with the realization of the nothingness at the heart of being comes deep anxiety.

Hence, though the term *freedom* is absent in therapy sessions and in psychotherapy manuals, its derivatives—responsibility, willing, wishing, deciding—are highly visible denizens of all psychotherapy endeavors.

CHAPTER 46

Helping Patients Assume Responsibility

As long as patients persist in believing that their major problems are a result of something outside their control—the actions of other people, bad nerves, social class injustices, genes—then we therapists are limited in what we can offer. We can commiserate, suggest more adaptive methods of responding to the assaults and unfairness of life; we can help patients attain equanimity, or teach them to be more effective in altering their environment.

But if we hope for more significant therapeutic change, we must encourage our patients to assume responsibility—that is, to apprehend how they themselves contribute to their distress. A patient may, for example, describe a series of horrendous experiences in the singles world: men mistreat her, friends betray her, employers exploit her, lovers deceive her. Even if the therapist is convinced of the veracity of the events described, there comes a time when attention must be paid to the patient's own role in the sequence of events. The therapist may have to say, in effect, "Even if ninety-nine percent of the bad things that happen to you is someone else's fault, I want to look at the other one percent—the part that is your responsibility. We have to look at your role, even if it's very limited, because that's where I can be of most help."

Readiness to accept responsibility varies greatly from patient to patient. Some arrive quickly at an understanding of their role in their discomfiture; others find responsibility assumption so difficult that it constitutes the major part of therapy, and once that step is taken, therapeutic change may occur almost automatically and effortlessly.

Every therapist develops methods to facilitate responsibility assumption. Sometimes I emphasize to a much-exploited patient that for every exploiter there must be an exploitee— that is, if they find themselves in an exploited role time and again, then surely the role must contain some lure for them. What might it be? Some therapists make the same point by confronting patients with the question, "What's the payoff for you in this situation?"

The group-therapy format offers particularly powerful leverage in helping patients comprehend their personal responsibility. Patients all begin the group together on equal footing and over the first weeks or months each member carves out a particular interpersonal role in the group—a role that is similar to the role each occupies in his/her outside life. Furthermore, the group is privy to how each member fashions that interpersonal role. These steps are far more obvious when tracked in the here-and-now than when the therapist tries to reconstruct them from the patient's own unreliable account.

The therapy group's emphasis on feedback initiates a responsibility-assumption sequence:

1. Members learn how their behavior is viewed by others;
2. Then they learn how their behavior makes others feel;

3. They observe how their behavior shapes others' opinions of them;
4. Finally, they learn that these first three steps shape the way they come to feel about themselves.

Thus the process begins with the patient's behavior and ends with the way each comes to be valued by others and by himself.

This sequence can form the base of powerful group therapist interventions. For example: "Joe, let's take a look at what is happening for you in the group. Here you are, after two months, not feeling good about yourself in this group and with several of the members impatient with you (or intimidated, or avoidant, or angry, or annoyed, or feeling seduced or betrayed). What's happened? Is this a familiar place for you? Would you be willing to take a look at your role in bringing this to pass?"

Individual therapists also take advantage of here-and-now data as they point out the patient's responsibility in the therapeutic process—for example, the patient's lateness, concealing information and feelings, forgetting to record dreams.

Responsibility assumption is an essential first step in the therapeutic process. Once individuals recognize their role in creating their own life predicament, they also realize that they, and only they, have the power to change that situation.

To look back over one's life and to accept the responsibility of what one has done to oneself may result in great regret. The therapist must anticipate that regret and attempt to reframe it. I often urge patients to project themselves into the future and to consider how they can live *now* so that five years hence they will be able to look back upon life without regret sweeping over them anew.

CHAPTER 47

Never (Almost Never)
Make Decisions for the Patient

Some years ago, Mike, a thirty-three-year-old physician, consulted me because of an urgent dilemma: he had a time-sharing condo in the Caribbean and planned to leave on vacation in one month. But there was a problem—a big problem. He had invited two women to accompany him and both had accepted—Darlene, his long-term girlfriend, and Patricia, a sparkling new woman he had met a couple of months before. What should he do? He was paralyzed with anxiety.

He described his relationship with the two women. Darlene, a journalist, had been the high school prom queen whom he had met again at a school reunion a few years ago. He found her beautiful and alluring, and fell in love with her on the spot. Though Mike and Darlene lived in different cities, they'd carried on an intense romance for the past three years, spoke daily on the phone, and spent most weekends and vacations together.

In the last several months, however, the ardor of the relationship had cooled. Mike felt less attracted to Darlene, their sex life languished, their phone conversations seemed desultory. Furthermore, her journalistic duties demanded so much travel that it was often difficult for her to get away for weekends and impossible for her to move closer to him. But Patricia, his new friend, seemed a dream come true: a pediatrician, elegant, wealthy, a half mile away, and most eager to be with him.

It seemed like a no-brainer. I reflected back to him his descriptions of the two women, wondering all the while, "What's the problem?" The decision seemed so obvious—Patricia was so right and Darlene so problematic—and the deadline so looming that I felt the strongest temptation to jump in and tell him to just get on with it and announce his decision, the only reasonable decision, that could possibly be made. What was the point of delay? Why make things worse for poor Darlene by cruelly and unnecessarily stringing her along?

Though I avoided the trap of telling him explicitly what to do, I managed to get my views across to him. We therapists have our little cunning ways—statements such as: "I wonder what blocks you from acting upon the decision you already seem to have made." (And I wonder, what on earth would therapists do without the device of "I wonder"?). And so in one way or another I did him the great service (in only three fast-paced sessions!) of mobilizing him into writing the inevitable "Dear John" letter to Darlene and sailing off into a glowing Caribbean sunset with Patricia.

But it didn't glow very long. Over the next several months strange things happened. Though Patricia continued to be a dream woman, Mike grew more uncomfortable at her insistence on closeness and commitment. He disliked her giving him the keys to her apartment and insisting that he reciprocate. And then, when Patricia suggested they live together, Mike balked. In our sessions he began to rhapsodize on how he treasured his space and solitude. Patricia was an extraordinary woman, without flaws. But he felt invaded. He did not want to live with her, or with anyone, and they soon drifted apart.

It was time for Mike to search for another relationship, and one day he showed me an ad he had posted in a computer-dating service. It specified particular characteristics of the woman he desired (beauty, loyalty, his approximate age and background) and described the type of relationship he was seeking (an exclusive but separate arrangement in which he and she would maintain their own space, speak often on the phone, and spend weekends and vacations together). "You know what, Doc," he said, wistfully, "sure sounds a lot like Darlene."

THE MORAL OF this cautionary tale is, beware of leaping in to make decisions for the patient. It is always a bad idea. As this vignette illustrates, not only do we lack a crystal ball, but we work with unreliable data. The information supplied by the patient is not only distorted but is likely to change as time passes or as the relationship with the therapist changes. Inevitably, new and unexpected factors emerge. If, as was true in this instance, the information the patient presents very strongly supports a specific course of action, then the patient, for any of a number of reasons, is seeking support for a particular decision that may or may not be the wisest course of action.

I have grown particularly skeptical of patients' accounts of spouses' culpability. Again and again I've had the experience of meeting the spouse and being astounded at the lack of convergence between the person in front of me and the person I have been hearing about for so many months. What generally gets omitted in accounts of marital discord is the patient's role in the process.

We are far better off relying on more reliable data—data not filtered through the patient's bias. There are two particularly useful sources of more objective observations: couples' sessions, where a therapist can view the interaction between partners, and focusing upon the here-and-now therapy relationship, in which therapists can view how patients contribute to their interpersonal relationships.

One caveat: There are times when the evidence of the patient's being abused by another is so strong—and the need for decisive action so clear—that it is incumbent upon the therapist to bring all possible influence to bear upon certain decisions. I do all that I can to discourage a woman with evidence of physical abuse from returning to a setting in which she is likely to be battered further. Hence the clause "Almost Never" in the title of this section.

Decisions: A *Via Regia* into Existential Bedrock

Leaping in to make decisions for patients is a good way to lose them. Patients assigned a task that they cannot or will not perform are unhappy patients. Whether they bridle at being controlled, or feel inadequate, or shudder at the prospect of disappointing their therapist, the result is often the same—they drop out of therapy.

But beyond the possibility of technical error is an even more pressing reason not to make decisions for patients: there is something much better to do with decision dilemmas. Decisions are a *via regia*, a royal road, into a rich existential domain—the realm of freedom, responsibility, choice, regret, wishing, and willing. To settle for superficial preemptive advice is to forgo the opportunity of exploring this realm with your patient.

Because decisional dilemmas ignite freedom-anxiety, many go to great lengths to steer clear of active decisions. That is why some patients seek delivery from decisions and, through cunning devices, inveigle unwary therapists to take the burden of decision away from them.

Or they force others in their life to make the decision for them: every therapist has seen patients who end relationships by so mistreating their partners that they will choose to leave. Others only hope for some overt transgression by the other: For example, one of my patients caught up in a highly destructive relationship said, "I can't bring myself to end this relationship, but I pray I could catch him in bed with another woman so that I would be able to leave him."

One of my first steps in therapy is to help patients assume responsibility for their actions. I try to help them understand that they make a decision even by not deciding or by maneuvering another into making a decision for them. Once patients accept that premise and own their behavior, then, in one manner or another, I pose the key therapy question: "Are you satisfied with that?" (Satisfied both with the nature of the decision and with their mode of making the decision.)

Take, for example, a married man having an affair who distances himself from his wife and so mistreats her that she, not he, makes the decision to end the marriage. I proceed by laying bare his pattern of disowning his decisions, a pattern that results in his feeling that he is controlled by external events. As long as he denies his own agency, real change is unlikely because his attention will be directed toward changing his environment rather than himself.

When this patient realizes his responsibility in ending the marriage and realizes also that it was he who chose to end it, then I turn his attention to how satisfied he is with *how* he made the decision. Did he act in good faith with his companion of so many years, with the mother of his children? What regrets will he have in the future? How much will he respect himself?

CHAPTER 49

Focus on Resistance to Decision

Why are decisions hard? In John Gardner's novel *Grendl*, the protagonist, confounded by life's mysteries, consults a wise priest who utters two simple phrases, four terrifying words: Everything fades and alternatives exclude.

"Alternatives exclude"—that concept lies at the heart of so many decisional difficulties. For every "yes" there must be a "no." Decisions are expensive because they demand renunciation. This phenomenon has attracted great minds throughout the ages. Aristotle imagined a hungry dog unable to choose between two equally attractive portions of food, and the medieval scholastics wrote of Burridan's ass, which starved to death between two equally sweet-smelling bales of hay.

In chapter 42 I described death as a boundary experience capable of moving an individual from an everyday state of mind to an ontological state (a state of being in which we are aware of being) in which change is more possible. Decision is another boundary experience. It not only confronts us with the degree to which we create ourselves but also to the limits of possibilities. Making a decision cuts us off from other possibilities. Choosing one woman, or one career, or one school, means relinquishing the possibilities of others. The more we face our limits, the more we have to relinquish our myth of personal specialness, unlimited potential, imperishability, and immunity to the laws of biological destiny. It is for these reasons that Heidegger referred to death as the *impossibility of further possibility.* The path to decision may be hard because it leads into the territory of both finiteness and groundlessness—domains soaked in anxiety. *Everything fades and alternatives exclude.*

CHAPTER 50

Facilitating Awareness by Advice Giving

Though we help patients deal with decision dilemmas primarily by helping them assume responsibility and by exposing the deep resistances to choosing, every therapist uses a number of other facilitating techniques.

Sometimes I offer advice or prescribe certain behaviors, *not as a way of usurping my patient's decision, but in order to shake up an entrenched thought or behavior pattern.* For example, Mike, a thirty-four-year-old scientist, agonized about whether he should stop in to visit his parents on an upcoming professional trip. Every time he had done that during the past few years he had, without fail, had a fight with his gruff blue-collar father, who resented having to meet him at the airport and berated him for not having rented a car.

His last trip had provoked such an acrimonious airport scene that he had cut his visit short and left without speaking again to his father. Yet he wanted to see his mother, with whom he was close and who agreed with him in his assessment of his father as a vulgar, insensitive cheapskate.

I urged Mike to visit his parents but to tell his father that he insisted on renting a car. Mike seemed shocked at my suggestion. His father had always met him at the airport—that was his role. Perhaps his father might be hurt at not being needed. Besides, why waste the money? He had no use for a car once he arrived at his parents' home. Why pay for it to sit there unused for a day or two?

I reminded him that his salary as a research scientist was more than double that of his father. And if he was worried about his father's being hurt, why not try having a gentle phone conversation with him, explaining the reasons for the car rental decision.

"A phone conversation with my father?" Mike said. "That's impossible. We never speak on the phone. I only speak to my mother when I phone."

"So many rules. So many fixed family rules," I mused. "You say you want things to change with your father? For that to happen, some family rules may have to be changed. What's the risk in opening everything up for discussion—on the phone, in person, even via a letter?"

The patient finally yielded to my exhortations and, in his own style and own voice, set about changing his relationship with his father. Changing one part of the family system always affects other parts, and in this instance his mother replaced his father as the chief family problem for several weeks. Eventually that too was resolved; the family gradually came together, and Mike had a keen sense of the role he had played in the distance that had existed between him and his father.

ANOTHER PATIENT, JARED, could not take the necessary steps to renew his green card. Though I knew there were potentially fertile dynamic issues underlying his procrastination, these would have to wait for us to explore because if he did not act immediately, he would be forced to leave the country, abandoning not only a promising research venture and a burgeoning romantic relationship, but therapy as well. I asked if he wanted my help with the green-card application.

He replied that he did and we charted out a course and schedule of action. He promised that, within twenty-four hours, he would e-mail me copies of his requests for letters of reference from former professors and employers and, at our next visit, seven days hence, he would bring his completed application to my office.

This intervention was sufficient to resolve the green-card crisis and permitted us then to turn our attention to the meaning of his procrastination, his feelings about my intervention, his wish for me to take over for him, and his need to be observed and succored.

ANOTHER EXAMPLE INVOLVES Jay, who wished to break off a relationship with Meg, a woman with whom he had been close for several years. She was a close friend to his wife and helped nurse her through a terminal illness and then supported him through a horrendous three-year bereavement. He had clung to Meg and lived with her during this time, but, as he recovered from his grief, he realized that they were not compatible and, after another painful year of indecision, he eventually asked her to move out.

Though he did not want her as a wife, he was exceedingly grateful to her and offered her a rent-free apartment in a building he owned. Thereafter he had a series of short-term relationships with women. Whenever one of these relationships ended, he was so agonized by isolation that he turned again to Meg until someone more suitable came alone. All the while he continued to give Meg slight hints that perhaps ultimately he and she might become a couple again. Meg responded by putting her life on hold and remaining in a state of perpetual readiness for him.

I suggested to him that his bad-faith actions with Meg were responsible not only for her being stuck in life, but also for much of his own low-grade dysphoria and guilt. He denied that he was acting in bad faith and cited as proof his largesse to Meg in offering her a rent-free apartment. If he really felt generous to her, I pointed out, why not provide for her in some manner that did not keep her bound to him—for example, give her an outright cash gift or the deed to a condo. A few more such confrontational sessions resulted in his acknowledging to himself and to me that he was selfishly refusing to let her go—he wanted to keep her on hold, as a backup, as insurance against loneliness.

IN EACH OF these instances the advice I offered was not meant to be an end in itself but a means to encourage exploration: into the rules of family systems, into the meaning and payoff of procrastination and dependent yearnings, into the nature and consequences of bad faith.

More often than not it is the process of giving advice that helps rather than the specific content of the advice. For example, a physician consulted me in a paralyzed state of procrastination. He was in serious trouble with his hospital because of his inability to complete medical charts, which resulted in a mountain of several hundred charts in his office.

I tried everything to mobilize him. I visited his office to appraise the magnitude of the task. I asked him to bring charts and a dictating machine to my office so that I could make suggestions about his dictation technique. We constructed a weekly schedule of dictation, and I phoned him to ascertain if he was sticking to it.

The content of none of these specific interventions was useful, but nonetheless he was moved by the process—that is, my caring enough to extend myself beyond the office space. The ensuing improvement in our relationship eventually led to good therapeutic work, resulting in his discovering his own methods to deal with his backlog.

CHAPTER 51

Facilitating Decisions—
Other Devices

L ike all therapists, I have favorite mobilizing techniques, developed over many years of practice. Sometimes I find it useful to underscore the absurdity of resistance based on past irreversible events. Once I had a resistive patient, very much stuck in life, who persisted in blaming his mother for events occurring decades previously. I helped him apprehend the absurdity of his position by asking him to repeat, several times, this statement: "I'm not going to change, Mother, till you treat me differently than when I was eight years old." From time to time, over the years I've used this device effectively (with variations in wording, of course, to fit a patient's particular situation). Sometimes I simply remind patients that sooner or later they will have to relinquish the goal of having a better past.

Other patients say they cannot act because they do not know what they want. In these instances, I try to help them locate and experience their wishes. This may be taxing, and ultimately many therapists grow weary and want to shout,

"Don't you ever want something?" Karen Horney sometimes said, perhaps in exasperation, "Have you ever thought to ask yourself what you want?" Some patients don't feel they have the right to want anything, others attempt to avoid the pain of loss by relinquishing wish. ("If I never wish, I will never again be disappointed.") Still others don't experience or express wishes in the hope that the grown-ups around them will divine their wants.

Occasionally individuals can recognize what they desire only when it is taken away from them. I've sometimes found it useful in working with individuals confused about their feelings about another to imagine (or to role-play) a telephone conversation in which the other breaks off the relationship. What do they feel then? Sadness? Hurt? Relief? Elation? Can we then find a way to allow these feelings to inform their proactive behavior and decisions?

Sometimes I've galvanized patients caught in a decisional dilemma by citing a line from Camus's *The Fall* that has always affected me deeply: "Believe me, the hardest thing for a man to give up is that which he really doesn't want, after all."

I've tried many ways to help patients see themselves more objectively. Sometimes a perspective-altering ploy I learned from a supervisor, Lewis Hill, is useful. I enlist the patient as a self-consultant in the following manner:

"Mary, I'm a bit stuck with one of my patients and I'd like your consultation; perhaps you might have some helpful suggestions. I'm seeing an intelligent, sensitive, attractive forty-five-year-old woman who tells me she is in an absolutely dreadful marriage. For years she had planned to leave her husband when her daughter went to college. That time has long come and gone and despite the fact that she is very unhappy she stays in the same situation. She says her husband is unloving and verbally abusive to her but she is unwilling to ask him to enter couples therapy, since she has decided to leave and if he changes in couples therapy that would be harder for her to do. But it is five years since her daughter left home and she is still there and things are still the same. She will neither enter marital therapy nor leave. I wonder whether she is wasting the only life she has in order to punish him. She says she wants him to make the move. She prays she could catch him in bed with another woman (or with a man—she has her suspicions about that), and that she would then be able to leave."

Of course, Mary quickly becomes aware that the patient is herself. Hearing herself described from a distance in third-person voice may permit her to gain more objectivity upon her situation.

CHAPTER 52

Conduct Therapy
as a Continuous Session

Many years ago I saw Rollo May in therapy over a two-year period. He lived and worked in Tiburon, I in Palo Alto, a seventy-five-minute drive away. I thought I might try to make good use of the commute by listening to a tape of the previous week's therapy session. Rollo agreed to my taping and I soon discovered that listening to the tape enhanced therapy wonderfully, since I plunged more quickly into deeper work on the important themes that had arisen in the previous session. So useful was it that, ever since, I have routinely taped sessions for patients who have a long commute to my office. Occasionally I do the same for patients who live nearby but have some peculiar inability to recall the previous session—perhaps great lability of affect or brief dissociative episodes.

This particular technique illustrates an important facet of therapy—namely that *therapy works best if it approximates a continuous session*. Therapy hours that are discontinuous from one to the next are far less effective. Using each therapy hour to solve the crises that have developed during the week is a particularly inefficient way to work. When I began in the field I heard David Hamburg, the chair of psychiatry at Stanford, refer jokingly to psychotherapy as "cyclotherapy," and indeed there is something to be said for that view in that we continually are engaged in "working through." We open up new themes, work on them for a while, move to other issues, but regularly and repetitively return to the same themes, each time deepening the inquiry. This cyclical aspect of the psychotherapy process has been compared to changing an automobile tire. We put the nuts on the bolt, tighten each evenly in turn until we return to the first, then repeat the process until the tire is optimally in place.

I am rarely the one who begins the session. Like most therapists, I prefer instead to wait for the patient. I want to know his or her "point of urgency" (as Melanie Klein referred to it). However, if I ever do open the session, it is invariably to refer back to the last meeting. Hence, if there was a particularly momentous or emotional or truncated session, I might begin, "We discussed many important things last week. I wonder what kind of feelings you took home with you."

My intent, of course, is to tie the current session into the last. My practice of writing summaries for the therapy group and mailing it to the group members before the next meeting serves exactly the same purpose. Sometimes groups begin with members taking issue with the summary. They point out that they saw things differently or that they now have an understanding different from the therapist's. I welcome the disagreement because it tightens the continuity of the sessions.

CHAPTER 53

Take Notes of Each Session

I f therapists are to be the historians of the therapy process and to attend to the continuity of the sessions, then it follows that they must keep some chronicle of events. Managed care and the threat of litigation, the twin plagues that today threaten the fabric of psychotherapy, have given us one positive gift: they have prompted therapists to take regular notes.

In the ancient times of secretaries I routinely dictated, and had transcribed, detailed summaries of each session. (Much of the material for this and other books is drawn from these notes.) Today, immediately after the hour, I take a few minutes to enter into the computer the major issues discussed in each session as well as my feelings and the unfinished business of each hour. I always arrange my schedule so that, without fail, I spend the necessary minutes to read the notes before the next session. If I find that there is nothing of significance to write, that in itself is an important piece of data and probably signifies that therapy is stagnating and the patient and I are breaking no new ground. Many therapists who see patients several times a week have less need for detailed notes because the sessions remain in mind more vividly.

CHAPTER 54

Encourage Self-Monitoring

The therapy venture is an exercise in self-exploration, and I urge patients to take advantage of any opportunity to sharpen our investigation. If a patient who has always been uncomfortable at social gatherings reports that he has received an invitation to a large party I usually respond, "Wonderful! What an opportunity to learn about yourself! Only this time monitor yourself—and be certain to jot down some notes afterward that we can discuss at the next session."

Visits home to parents are particularly rich sources of information. At my suggestion many of my patients begin to have longer and deeper conversations with siblings than ever before. And any type of class reunion is generally a gold mine of data, as are any opportunities to revisit old relationships. I urge patients also to attempt to obtain feedback from others about how they were or are perceived. I know one elderly man who met someone from his fifth-grade class who told him that she remembered him as a "beautiful boy with coal-black hair and a sly smile." He wept as he heard that. He had always regarded himself as homely and awkward. Had someone, anyone, only told him *then* that he was beautiful, it would have, he believed, changed his whole life.

CHAPTER 55

When Your Patient Weeps

What do you do when a friend weeps in your presence? Ordinarily you attempt to offer comfort. "There, there," you might say consolingly, or you may hold your friend, or rush for tissues, or search for some way to help your friend regain control and stop weeping. The therapy situation, however, calls for something beyond comforting.

Because weeping often signifies the entry into deeper chambers of emotion, the therapist's task is not to be polite and help the patient stop weeping. Quite the contrary—you may wish to encourage your patients to plunge even deeper. You may simply urge them to share their thoughts: "Don't try to leave that space. Stay with it. Please keep talking to me; try to put your feelings into words." Or you may ask a question I often use: "If your tears had a voice, what would they be saying?"

Psychotherapy may be thought of as an *alternating sequence of affect expression and affect analysis*. In other words, you encourage acts of emotional expression but you always follow with reflection upon the emotions expressed. This sequence is far more evident in group therapy because such strong emotions are evoked in a group setting, but it is also evident in the individual setting, particularly in the act of weeping. Hence, when weeping occurs I first plunge the patient into the content and meaning of the weeping and later make sure to analyze the act of weeping, especially insofar as it relates to the here-and-now. Hence, I inquire not only into feelings about weeping in general but, in particular, how it feels to weep *in my presence*.

CHAPTER 56

Give Yourself Time
Between Patients

I expect this unpopular tip to be passed over quickly by many therapists whose practice is swept along by the swift current of economic necessity, but here goes anyway.

Don't shortchange yourself and the patient by not leaving ample time between sessions. I have always kept detailed notes of each session and I never begin a session without referring to them. My notes often indicate the unfinished business—themes and topics that should be pursued or feelings between me and the patient that were not fully worked through. If you take each hour seriously, then the patient will as well.

Some therapists schedule so tightly that they have no break whatsoever between patients. Even ten minutes is, in my view, insufficient if a good chunk of that time is spent returning calls. I never take less than a full ten minutes and prefer fifteen minutes for note taking, note reading, and thinking between patients. Fifteen-minutes intervals pose complications: patients must be scheduled at odd times—for example, ten minutes before or after the hour—but all my patients have taken this in stride. It also lengthens your day and may diminish income. But it is worth it. Abraham Lincoln is reputed to have said that if he had eight hours to cut down a tree, he'd spend several of these hours sharpening his ax. Don't become the woodcutter who is too rushed to sharpen the ax.

CHAPTER 57

Express Your Dilemmas Openly

Generally when I am stuck and have difficulty responding to a patient, it is because I am caught between two or more competing considerations. I believe you can almost never go wrong by expressing your dilemma openly. Some examples follow.

"Ted, let me interrupt. I feel a bit caught today between two opposing feelings: on the one hand I know that the history of your conflict with your boss is important and I know, too, that often you feel hurt when I interrupt you; but on the other hand I have the strongest sense of your avoiding something important today."

"Mary, you say you don't believe I'm being fully honest with you, that I'm too tactful and delicate with you. I think you're right: I do hold back. I often feel caught in a dilemma: on the one hand I wish to be more natural with you and yet, on the other hand, because I feel that you're easily wounded and that you give my comments inordinate power, I feel I must consider my wording very, very carefully."

"Pete, I've got a dilemma. I know Ellie is the topic you want to discuss with me: I sense your strong press to do so and I don't want to frustrate you. But on the other hand you say you know your relationship with her makes no sense, that it is all wrong for you, that it will never work out. It seems to me that we've got to go beneath or beyond Ellie and try to discover more of what fuels your powerful infatuation. Your descriptions of the details of your interaction with Ellie have taken up so much of our recent hours that we've little time for deeper exploration. I suggest we limit the time we discuss Ellie—perhaps to ten minutes each session."

"Mike, I don't want to avoid your question. I know you feel I duck your personal inquiries. I don't want to do that and I promise to come back to your questions. But I do feel it would be more helpful to our work if we first looked at all the reasons behind your questions."

One final example. Susan was a patient who came to see me when she was on the verge of leaving her husband. After several months of productive therapy she felt better and had improved her relationship with her husband. One session she described a recent conversation with her husband during lovemaking in which she mimicked a statement of mine (distorting it as well), which provided them a good belly laugh. The joint mocking of me served to bring them closer together.

How to respond? I had a number of possibilities. First, this event reflected how close she felt to her husband—the closest they had been for a very long time, perhaps years. We had been working hard toward this end, and I could have expressed some of my pleasure at her progress. Or I might have responded to her distortion of my remark to him. Or I might have commented on how she handled triangles in general—she had a well-established pattern of great unease in three-way relationships, including the oedipal triangle—she, her husband, and son; she and two friends; and now she, her husband, and me. But my overriding feeling was that she had treated me in bad faith, and I didn't like it. I knew that she had much gratitude and many positive feelings toward me but, nonetheless, she had chosen to trivialize her relationship with me in order to augment her relationship with her husband. But was this feeling justified? Was I not putting my personal pique in the way of what was professionally best for the patient?

Ultimately, I decided to disclose each of these feelings and my dilemma about revealing them. My disclosure led us into a fruitful discussion of several important issues. She grasped immediately that our triangle was a microcosm and that other friends of hers must have experienced feelings similar to mine. Yes, it was true that her husband felt threatened by me and that she wanted to soothe him by mocking me. But perhaps was it also true that she had unconsciously fanned his competitive feelings? And was there no way for her to offer him some genuine reassurance and at the same time maintain the integrity of her relationship with me? My giving voice to my feelings opened up an inquiry into her entrenched and maladaptive pattern of playing one person off against the other.

CHAPTER 58

Do Home Visits

I have paid a few home calls on my patients. Far too few—for, without exception, each one has proven profitable. Each visit has informed me about aspects of my patients that I would have never otherwise known—their hobbies, the intrusiveness of their work, their aesthetic sensibility (evidenced by the furnishings, decorations, artworks), their recreational habits, evidence of books and magazines in the home. One patient who complained of his lack of friends had a particularly unkempt home that showed little sensitivity to the sensibilities of visitors. A young, attractive, well-groomed woman who sought help because of her inability to form good relationship with men showed such little care about her home surroundings—heavily stained carpets, a dozen cardboard boxes full of old mail, tattered furniture—that it was not surprising to me that her male visitors were turned off.

In a home visit to another patient I learned for the first time that she kept over a dozen cats and that her house so reeked of cat urine that she could never entertain in her home. A visit to the home of a brusque, insensitive man contained, to my wonderment, walls covered with examples of his exquisite Chinese landscapes and calligraphy.

The discussion preceding the home visit may be particularly productive. Patients may develop anxiety about such exposure; they may vacillate about whether they should do a housecleaning or allow their home to be viewed au naturel. One patient grew very anxious and resisted my visit for some time. When I saw her apartment she appeared exceedingly embarrassed as she showed me a wall covered with mementos of past lovers: carnival dolls, opera ticket stubs, Tahiti and Acapulco snapshots. Her embarrassment? She had a strong desire to win my respect for her intellectual ability and was ashamed of my seeing her so imprisoned by the past. She knew that it was foolish to be eternally mooning about her past loves and felt that I would be disappointed in her when I saw how heavily she encumbered herself.

Another patient in deep grief spoke so often of the presence of his wife's effects and photographs that I suggested a home visit and found his house to be filled with material reminders of his wife, including, in the middle of the living room, the old, shabby sofa upon which she had died. The walls were covered by her photographs, either of her or photographs that she had taken, and by bookcases filled with her books. Most important of all: there was so little of him in the house—his taste, his interests, his comforts! The visit proved meaningful to the patient in terms of process—that I cared enough to extend myself to make the visit—and it ushered in a stage of dramatic change as he declared he wanted my help in changing his home. Together we worked out a schedule and approach to a series of home alterations that both facilitated and reflected progress in the grief work.

Still others showed little caring about themselves, as though they deserved no beauty, no comfort, in their lives. One patient, much to my surprise, proved to be a hoarder with hundreds of old magazines and phone books in heaps around the house—a fact I might never have otherwise learned. A patient of one of my students who was also a hoarder finally agreed after two years of therapy to a visit by the therapist with these words: "You have to promise not to cry." Her comment suggests that her permission for the visit was an indication that she had genuinely begun the process of change.

Home visits are significant events, and I do not intend to convey that beginning therapists undertake such a step lightly. Boundaries first need to be established and respected, but when the situation requires it, we must be willing to be flexible, creative, and individualized in the therapy we offer. On the other hand, however, one wonders why the tradition of home visiting, once so common in health care, now seems so bold and risky. I am glad to see the changes now occurring, beginning with family therapists who more often make a point of scheduling sessions in their patients' homes.

CHAPTER 59

Don't Take Explanation
Too Seriously

In an experiment I described earlier, in which a patient and I each recorded our views of each therapy session, I learned that we remembered and valued very different aspects of the process. I valued my intellectual interpretations whereas these made little impact on the patient, who valued instead the small personal acts relevant to our relationship. Most published firsthand accounts of psychotherapy point to the same discrepancy: *Therapists place a far higher value than patients on interpretation and insight.* We therapists grossly overvalue the content of the intellectual treasure hunt; it has been this way from the very beginning, when Freud got us off to a bad start with two of his enticing but misguided metaphors.

The first was the image of the therapist-cum-archaeologist painstakingly brushing the dust off buried memories to uncover the truth—what really happened in the patient's early years: the original trauma, the primal scene, the primordial events. The second metaphor was that of the jigsaw puzzle. Find only the last missing piece, Freud suggested, and the entire puzzle will be solved. Many of his case histories read like mysteries, and readers eagerly push ahead, anticipating a juicy denouement in which all riddles will find their solution.

Naturally we convey our enthusiasm for the intellectual hunt to our patients, and we observe or imagine their "aha" reactions to our interpretations. Nietzsche said, "We even invent the expression on the face of the other with whom we converse to coincide with the brilliant thought we think we have uttered." Freud took no pains to conceal his enthusiasm for intellectual solutions. More than one of his former patients have described his habit of reaching for his box of "Victory cigars" to celebrate a particularly incisive interpretation. And the popular media have long presented this mistaken view of therapy to the public. Hollywood characteristically portrays psychotherapists lurching through many obstacles, following many wrong trails, overcoming lust and danger to arrive ultimately at the great clarifying and redemptive insight.

I do not mean that the intellectual venture is not important. Indeed it is, but not for the reasons we usually think. We crave the comfort of absolute truth because we cannot bear the desolation of a purely capricious existence. As Nietzsche put it, "Truth is an illusion without which a certain species could not survive." Anointed, as we are, with an inbuilt solution-seeking, gestalt-filling need, we cling tenaciously to the belief that explanation, some explanation, is possible. It makes things bearable, it anoints us with a sense of control and mastery.

But it is not the *content* of the intellectual treasure trove that matters but the *hunt*, which is the perfect therapy mating task, offering something to each participant: Patients bask in the attention paid to the most minute details of their life, and the therapist is entranced by the process of solving the riddle of a life. The beauty of it is that it keeps patient and therapist tightly connected while the real agent of change—*the therapeutic relationship*—is germinating.

In practice, there is a great complexity in the link between the intellectual project and the therapist-patient relationship. The more that therapists know about the patient's life, past and present, the more they enter into it and become a closer and more sympathetic witness. Furthermore, many interpretations are explicitly directed toward improving the therapist-patient relationship—repeatedly therapists focus upon identifying and clarifying the obstacles blocking the encounter between themselves and their patient.

At the most fundamental level the relationship between insight and change remains an enigma. Though we take for granted that insight leads to change, by no means is that sequence established empirically. In fact there are experienced, thoughtful analysts who have raised the possibility of a reversed sequence—that is, that insight *follows* change rather than precedes it.

And, finally, bear in mind Nietzsche's dictum: "There is no truth, there is only interpretation." Hence, even if we do offer some elegantly packaged insight of extraordinary we must realize it is a construct, *an* explanation, not *the* explanation.

Consider a despairing widow who could not tolerate being alone and unpaired but nonetheless sabotaged any potential new relationship with a man. Why? Over several months of investigation we arrived at several explanations:

- She feared that she was cursed. Every man she had loved met an untimely end. She avoided intimacy in order to protect the man from her bad karma.

- She feared a man's getting too close because he would be able to see into her and discover her fundamental badness, smuttiness, and murderous rage.

- If she really permitted herself to love another it would be a final acknowledgment that her husband was indeed dead.

- Loving another man would constitute treason: it would signify that her love for her husband was not as deep as she had thought.

- She had had too many losses and could not survive another one. Men were too frail; whenever she looked at a new man in her life, she saw his skull gleaming under his skin and was besieged by thoughts about his soon becoming a bag of dry bones.

- She hated to face her own helplessness. There were times when her husband got angry with her and she would be devastated by his anger. She was determined not to let that ever happen again, never to give anyone that much control over her.

- Settling for one man meant giving up the possibility of any other man, and she was loath to relinquish her possibilities.

Which of these explanations was true, was the correct one? One? Some? All? Each represents a different construct: there are as many explanations as there are explanatory systems. None at the time proved to make the crucial difference. But the search for explanation kept us engaged and our engagement ultimately made the difference. She took the plunge and chose to relate deeply to me, and I did not shrink away from her. I was not destroyed by her rage, I remained close to her, I held her hand when she was most despairing, I stayed alive and did not fall victim to her cursed karma.

CHAPTER 60

Therapy-Accelerating Devices

Therapy or personal-growth groups have, for decades, used accelerating, or "unfreezing," techniques. Some that I have found useful include the "trust fall," in which the group forms a circle around a member who, eyes closed, falls backward to be caught by the group members. In the "top secret" exercise, each of the members writes down, on uniform slips of paper without identifying details, a top secret that would feel risky for them to reveal. The statements are then redistributed and each member reads someone else's top secret and discusses how she would feel if she had such a secret. Another technique is to play back selected sections of the videotape of a previous meeting. Or, in student groups, members alternate the role of the group leader and critique one another's performance. Or, to break a long initial silence, the leader may suggest a rapid "go-around" in which members reveal some of their free associations during the silence.

All of these unfreezing, or accelerating, techniques *are only the first stage of the exercise*. In each instance the group leader must debrief, must help the group members harvest the data generated by the exercise: for example, their attitudes toward trust, empathy, and self-disclosure.

One of the most powerful interventions I have used (in groups of cancer patients as well as in a didactic setting for large audiences) is the "Who am I?" exercise. Each member is given eight slips of paper and instructed to write an answer to "Who am I?" on each slip. (Some likely answers: a wife, a female, a Christian, a lover of books, a mother, a physician, an athlete, a sexual being, an accountant, an artist, a daughter, etc.). Then each member arranges the slips in order from most peripheral to most central (that is, closest to one's core).

After that, the members are instructed to meditate upon a slip, beginning with the most peripheral, and to imagine what it would feel like to let go of that part of one's identity. A signal (a soft bell or chime) every couple of minutes moves them to the next slip, and after the bell chimes eight times and all the slips have been covered, the procedure is reversed and the members reappropriate each of the aspects of their identity. In the post-exercise discussion (essential in this exercise as in all others), the members discuss the issues evoked for them: for example, issues of identity and core self, the experience of letting go, fantasies about death.

In general, I find such accelerating devices less necessary or useful in individual therapy. Some approaches to therapy—for example, gestalt therapy—use a great many exercises that, if used judiciously, may facilitate therapy. But it is also true that some young therapists err by developing a grab bag of exercises and reach into it to jazz up therapy whenever it seems to have slowed down. Beginning therapists must learn that there are times to sit in silence, sometimes in silent communion, sometimes simply while waiting for patients' thoughts to appear in a form that may be expressed.

However, in accord with the dictum that one must invent a different therapy for each patient, there are appropriate times for a therapist to develop some exercise that fits the needs of a particular patient.

Elsewhere in this text I discuss a number of such devices: a home visit, role playing, or asking patients to compose their epitaph. I also ask patients to bring in old family photos. Not only do I feel more linked to the patient when I share some of their images of past important figures, but the patient's memory of significant past events and feelings is greatly catalyzed by the old photos. Occasionally it is useful to ask patients to write a letter (to be shared with me and not necessarily to be mailed) to someone with whom they may have important unfinished business—for example, an unavailable or dead parent, an ex-wife, a child.

The most common technique I use is informal role playing. If, for example, a patient discusses her inability to confront a partner about some issue—let's say that she is anxious about a weeklong seaside vacation with a friend because she needs to have time off each day to be alone to meditate, to read, or to think. I might suggest a brief role-play exercise in which she plays her friend and I take her role to demonstrate how she might make such a request. On other occasions I might do the opposite: play the other person and have her practice what she might say.

Fritz Perls's empty-chair technique is sometimes useful. I instruct some patients with a strong self-deprecatory inner voice to put the judging, self-critical part of them in an empty chair and speak to it, then to change chairs and play the judge expressing the critical comments to the manifest self. Again, I emphasize, such techniques are useful not as ends in themselves, but to generate data for subsequent exploration.

CHAPTER 61

Therapy as a Dress Rehearsal
for Life

Many therapists cringe when they hear critics charac-
terize their work as merely the "purchase of friendship." Though there is a grain of truth in this
statement, it does not merit a cringe. Friendship between therapist and patient is a necessary condition in the process of therapy—*necessary, but not, however, sufficient*. Psychotherapy is
not a substitute for life but a dress rehearsal for life. In other
words, though psychotherapy requires a close relationship, the
relationship is not an end—it is a means to an end.

The closeness of the therapy relationship serves many purposes. It affords a safe place for patients to reveal themselves as
fully as possible. More than that, it offers them the experience
of being accepted and understood after deep disclosure. It
teaches social skills: The patient learns what an intimate relationship requires. And the patient learns that intimacy is possible, even achievable. Lastly, and perhaps most important of all,
is Carl Rogers's observation that the therapy relationship serves
as an internal reference point to which patients can return in

their imagination. Having once achieved this level of intimacy, they can harbor the hope and even the expectation of similar relationships.

One often hears of patients (in either group therapy or individual therapy) who are excellent patients or group members, yet remain essentially unchanged in their external lives. They may relate well to the individual therapist or may be key members of groups—self-disclosing, working hard, catalyzing interaction—and yet do not apply what they have learned to their outside situation. In other words, they use therapy as a substitute rather than a rehearsal for life.

This distinction may prove useful in termination decisions. Behavior change in the therapy situation is obviously not enough: patients must transfer their change into their life environment. In the late stages of therapy, I am energetic in ensuring transfer of learning. If I deem it necessary, I begin to coach actively, to press the patient to experiment with new behaviors in work, social, and family settings.

CHAPTER 62

Use the Initial Complaint as Leverage

Don't lose touch with patients' initial complaints. As the following vignette illustrates, the reasons for seeking therapy given in the first session may serve you in good stead during difficult phases of therapy.

A FIFTY-FIVE-YEAR-OLD FEMALE therapist sought my consultation because of an impasse in her work with Ron, a forty-year-old clinical psychology student whom she had been seeing for a few months. A short time before, Ron had been rejected by a woman he had dated a few times, and thereafter he grew more demanding in the therapy hours and insisted that his therapist hold his hand and give him comforting hugs. To support his case he brought in a copy of my book *Momma and the Meaning of Life,* in which I described the salubrious effects of holding the hand of a grieving widow. Ron pouted, refused to shake hands at the end of sessions, and drew up lists of his therapist's shortcomings.

The therapist felt increasingly uncomfortable, confused,

manipulated, and annoyed with Ron's infantile behavior. Every approach she had made to ameliorate the impasse had failed, and, growing frightened at the depth of her patient's anger, she was contemplating terminating therapy.

In supervision we reviewed Ron's initial reason for seeking therapy—to work on his relationships with women. An attractive man who formed relationships with women easily, Ron spent most evenings with his barroom chums picking up women for one-night stands and quickly moving on to others. On those few occasions when he found a woman particularly attractive, and wished to continue the relationship, he had been dumped precipitously. He wasn't sure why but he guessed that she had gotten fed up with his insistence that he get exactly what he wanted at all times. It was precisely because of these issues that he had selected a female therapist.

This information shed much light on the therapy impasse and provided important leverage. The contretemps between the patient and therapist was no unfortunate complication in therapy, it was an inevitable and essential development. *Of course* Ron would demand too much from his therapist. *Of course* he would demean her, and *of course* she would wish to leave him. But how to turn that to therapeutic use?

Remember chapter 40, "Feedback: Strike When the Iron Is Cold." Timing is all-important: interpretations are most effective when the patient's affect has sufficiently diminished to permit him to assume a more dispassionate view of his behavior. When that time arrives, use the leverage afforded by the presenting problem. Bank on the therapeutic alliance and suggest that therapist and patient together attempt to understand the course of events. For example:

> "Ron, I think what's been happening between us the last few weeks is really important. Let me tell you why.

Think back on the reasons you first came to see me. It was because of problems that persistently arose between you and women. Given that, it was inevitable that uncomfortable issues would arise between the two of us. And that has come to pass. So, even though this is not comfortable for you—nor for me—we should still regard it as an unusual learning opportunity. Things have happened here that are reflective of what happens in your social life, but there is one fundamental difference—and that's what is unique about the therapy situation: *I'm not going to break off contact and I'm going to be available for you to find out something you've never been privy to in past relationships—the feelings evoked in the other person by your actions.*"

Following this, the therapist may proceed to share the feelings she has about Ron's behavior, taking care to frame them gently and supportively.

CHAPTER 63

Don't Be Afraid of Touching Your Patient

A t the onset of my psychiatry training at Johns Hopkins, I attended an analytic case conference at which a discussant soundly criticized the young therapist presenting a case because he helped his patient (an elderly woman) put on her overcoat at the end of a session. A long, heated debate followed. Some less judgmental members of the conference agreed that, though it was obvious the therapist had erred, the patient's advanced age and the raging snowstorm outside lessened the gravity of the offense.

I've never forgotten that conference and even now, decades later, a fellow resident with whom I have remained friends and I still joke about the overcoat caper and the inhumane view of therapy it represented. It took years of practice and remedial experiences to undo the damage of such rigid training.

One such remedial experience occurred while I was developing methods of leading support groups for patients with cancer. After my first group had been meeting a few months, a member suggested a different way to end the meeting. She lit a candle, asked us to join hands, then led the group in a guided meditation. I had never held hands with a patient before but in this situation I had no choice. I joined in and immediately felt, like all the members, that it was an inspired way to end our meetings, and for several years we closed each session in this manner. The meditation was calming and restorative but it was the touching of hands that particularly moved me. Artificial boundaries—patient and therapist, the sick and the well, the dying and the living—evaporated as we all felt joined to the others by a common humanity.

I make a point to touch each patient each hour—a hand-shake, a clasp of the shoulder, usually at the end of the hour as I accompany the patient to the door. If a patient wants to hold my hand longer or wants a hug, I refuse only if there is some compelling reason—for example, concerns about sexual feel-ings. But, whatever the contact, I make a point to debrief at the next session—perhaps something as simple as: "Mary, our last hour ended differently—you held on to my hand with both of yours for a long time [or "You asked for a hug"]. It seemed to me that you were feeling something strongly. What can you remember of it?" I believe that most therapists have their own secret rules about touching. Decades ago, for example, an eld-erly, particularly skilled therapist told me that for many years her patients routinely ended the session by kissing her on the cheek.

Do touch. But make sure the touch becomes grist for the interpersonal mill.

If a patient is in great despair because of, let us say, a cancer recurrence or any other awful life event and asks during the ses-sion to hold my hand or for a hug, I would no sooner refuse than to decline to help an old woman facing a snowstorm put on her overcoat. If I can find no way to ease the pain, I may ask what he/she would like from me that day—to sit in silence, to ask questions and more actively guide the sessions? To move my chair closer? To hold hands? To the best of my ability, I try to respond in a loving, human way, but later, as always, I debrief: I talk about what feelings my actions produced, and I share my feelings as well. If I have a concern that my actions may be interpreted as sexual, then I share those concerns openly and make it clear that, though sexual feelings may be experienced in the therapy relationship and should be expressed and discussed, they will never be acted upon. Nothing takes precedence, I emphasize, over the importance of the patient's feeling safe in the therapy office and the therapy hour.

I never, of course, press contact. If, for example, a patient leaves in anger, refusing a handshake, I immediately respect that wish for distance. More deeply troubled patients may at times experience powerful and idiosyncratic feelings about touch, and if I am uncertain of those feelings, I make explicit inquiry. "Shall we shake hands as usual today? Or is it best, today, not to?" In all of these instances I invariably examine the incident the following session.

These general points serve as a beacon in therapy. Dilemmas about touch in therapy are not common, but when they occur it is important that therapists not be fettered by legalistic concerns and be able, as the following example demonstrates, to be responsive, responsible, and creative in their work.

A middle-aged woman I had been seeing for a year had lost most of her hair because of radiotherapy for a brain tumor. She was preoccupied by her appearance and often remarked how hideous others would find her without her wig. I asked how she thought I would react. She felt that I, too, would change my views of her and would find her so repellent that I would shrink away from her. I opined that I could not imagine shrinking away from her.

In the weeks following she entertained thoughts of removing her wig in my office, and at one session she announced that the time had come. She gulped and, after asking me to look away, removed her wig and, with the aid of her pocket mirror, arranged her remaining wisps of hair. When I turned my gaze back to her, I had a moment, only a moment, of shock at how she had suddenly aged, but I quickly reconnected with the essence of the lovely person I knew and entertained a fantasy of running my fingers through her wisps of hair. When she asked about my feelings, I shared the fantasy. Her eyes flooded with tears and she reached for the Kleenex. I decided to push further. "Shall we try it?" I asked. "That would be a wonderful thing," she replied, and so I moved next to her and stroked her hair and scalp. Though the experience lasted for only a few moments, it remained indelible in both of our minds. She survived her cancer and, years later, when she returned because of another issue, she remarked that my touching her scalp had been an epiphany, an immensely affirming action that radically changed her negative image of herself.

A similar testimonial came from a widow who was in such despair that she often came to my office too distressed to speak, but was deeply comforted sheerly by my holding her hand. Much later she remarked that it was a turning point in therapy: it had grounded her and allowed her to feel connected to me. My hand, she said, was ballast preventing her from drifting up and away into despair.

CHAPTER 64

Never Be Sexual with Patients

The high incidence of sexual transgressions has become a grave problem over the past few years, not only in psychotherapy, of course, but in all situations in which a power differential exists: the priesthood, the military, the corporate and political workplace, medicine, educational institutions—you name it. Though such transgressions constitute a momentous problem in each of these settings, they have particular meaning in the field of psychotherapy, in which intense and intimate relationships are so essential to the endeavor and in which sexual relationships are so destructive to all parties, therapists as well as patients.

Psychotherapy is doubly cursed by such transgressions. Not only are individual patients betrayed and damaged, but the resulting backlash has been highly destructive for the whole field. Therapists have been forced to practice defensively. Professional organizations instruct practitioners to exercise extreme caution. They are warned not only against any unusual intimacy but against any semblance of intimacy, because the legal profession assumes that where there is smoke there must be fire. In other words, we are advised to adopt a "snapshot" mentality—that is, avoid any moment that, taken even out of context, might appear suspicious. Avoid informality, therapists are told; avoid first names, do not offer coffee or tea, do not run over the fifty-minute hour, and do not see a member of the opposite sex for the last hour of the day (all offenses to which I plead guilty). Some clinics have considered videotaping all sessions to ensure the safety of patients. I know a therapist who, once sued unjustly, now refuses any physical contact, even a handshake, with patients.

These are dangerous developments. If we don't regain balance in this area, we will sacrifice the very core of psychotherapy. It is for this reason that I wrote the previous tip on touching. And it is to ensure that the student not fall into the error of equating therapeutic intimacy and sexual intimacy that I hasten now to offer the following comments on sexual transgression.

Strong sexual feelings haunt the therapy situation. How could they not, given the extraordinary intimacy between patient and therapist? Patients regularly develop feelings of love and/or sexual feelings for their therapist. The dynamics of such positive transference are often overdetermined. For one thing, patients are exposed to a very rare, gratifying, and delicious situation. Their every utterance is examined with interest, every event of their past and present life is explored, they are nurtured, cared for, and unconditionally accepted and supported.

Some individuals do not know how to respond to such generosity. What can they offer in return? Many women, especially those with low self-regard, believe that the only real gift they have to offer is a sexual gift. Without sex—a commodity they may have depended upon in past relationships—they can only foresee a loss of interest and ultimate abandonment by the therapist. For others, who elevate the therapist to an unrealistic, lofty, larger-than-life position, there may also be the wish to merge with something greater than themselves. Still others may compete for love with the unknown patients in the therapist's practice.

All of these dynamics should become part of the therapy dialogue: they have in one way or another created difficulty for the patient in his/her life, and it is good, not unfortunate, that they emerge in the here-and-now of the therapy hour. Since attraction to the therapist is to be expected, this phenomenon, like all events in the therapy hour, should be explicitly addressed and understood. If therapists find themselves aroused by the patient, that very arousal constitutes data about the patient's way of being (assuming the therapist is clear about his/her own reactions).

Therapists do not gratify masochistic patients by beating them. Neither should he or she become sexually involved with patients who crave sex. Although the majority of sexual transgressions occur between a male therapist and a female patient (for this reason I use "he" for the therapist in this discussion), similar issues and temptations apply for female and for gay therapists.

Therapists who have a history of feeling unattractive to women may be exhilarated and destabilized when avidly sought after by female patients. Keep in mind that the feelings arising in the therapy situation generally belong more to the role than the person: Do not mistake the transferential adoration as a sign of your irresistible personal attractiveness or charm.

Some therapists run into difficulty because they have an unfulfilled sexual life or live in too much isolation to make the appropriate and necessary sexual contacts. Obviously, it is a grave error to look to one's practice as an opportunity for such contacts. It is important for therapists to do whatever is necessary to correct their situation—be that individual therapy, marital therapy, dating services, computer matching, you name it. When I meet with such therapists in therapy or supervision I want to tell them, and often do, that *any* option, including visiting a prostitute, is preferable to the calamitous choice of acting out sexually with patients; I want to tell them, and often do, to find some way of fulfilling their sexual needs with one of the billions of potential partners in the world: anyone except their patients. That is simply not a professional or moral option.

If, in the final analysis, the therapist can find no solution to unruly sexual impulses and is unable or unwilling to get help from personal therapy, then I believe he should not be practicing psychotherapy.

Sexual transgression is also destructive for therapists. Offending therapists, once they examine themselves honestly, understand that they are acting for their own satisfaction rather than in the service of their patient. Therapists who have made a deep commitment to a life of service do great violence to themselves and to their innermost moral precepts. They ultimately pay a devastatingly high price not only from the external world in the form of civil censure and punishment and widespread disapprobation, but internally as well, in the form of pervasive and persistent shame and guilt.

CHAPTER 65

Look for Anniversary and Life-Stage Issues

Certain dates may have great significance for many patients. As a result of many years of working with bereaved individuals, I have grown to respect the persistence and power of anniversary reactions. Many bereaved spouses feel buffeted by sudden waves of despair that coincide with milestones of their spouse's demise—for example, the date of definitive diagnosis, the death, or the funeral. Not infrequently, the patient is consciously unaware of the precise dates—a phenomenon that has always seemed to me a persuasive proof, if one is needed, of the existence of unconscious influence upon conscious thoughts and feelings. Such anniversary reactions may recur unabated in power for years, even decades. The professional literature contains many startling studies documenting the anniversary reaction, such as the increased incidence of psychiatric hospitalization on the anniversaries, even decades later, of parental death days.

Certain notable dates provide openings for therapy inquiry in a multitude of ways. Birthdays, especially significant birthdays, may provide an open window to existential concerns and lead to an increased contemplation of the life cycle. In adulthood, birthday celebrations are always, it seems to me, bittersweet affairs with an underside of lament. Some individuals are affected by a birthday that signifies outliving their parents. Dates of retirement, wedding or divorce anniversaries, and many other markers bring home to the individual the inexorable march of time and the transience of life.

CHAPTER 66

Never Ignore "Therapy Anxiety"

Although I stress that psychotherapy is a creative and spontaneous process shaped by each practitioner's unique style and customized for each patient, there are, nonetheless, certain universal rules. One such rule is *always explore session-related anxiety*. If a patient experiences anxiety during the session, after the session (on the way home or later while thinking about the hour), or when preparing to come to the next session, then I always make a point of focusing in depth upon that anxiety.

Although the anxiety may sometimes issue from the *content* of the therapy discussion, far more commonly it stems from the *process*—from feelings about the patient-therapist relationship.

For example, one patient described feeling anxious entering my office:

"Why? What makes you anxious about coming here?" I asked.

"I'm frightened. I feel I'm skating on thin ice here."

"What is the equivalent of falling through the ice in our therapy?"

"That you'll be sick of my complaining and moaning and not want to see me again."

"That must complicate things for you a great deal. I tell you to express all your troubling thoughts. That's hard enough, but then you add to it something else—that you must also take care not to burden or discourage me."

Or another patient:

"I didn't want to come today. I've been upset all week about what you said to me when I took the Kleenex."

"What did you hear me say?"

"That you were fed up with me complaining and not accepting your help."

"What I remember was something very different. You were weeping and, wanting to comfort you, I reached to offer you a Kleenex. I was struck by how quickly you moved to take it yourself—as though to avoid taking something from me—and tried to encourage you to explore your feelings about taking help from me. But that's by no means the same as a criticism or being 'fed up.'"

"I do have some feelings about taking help from you. I think of you as having a finite amount of caring—only one hundred points—and I don't want to use up all my points."

If a patient develops anxiety *during* the session, I become a detective and enlist the patient's aid in going over the session microscopically to determine precisely when the discomfort arose. The process of such an inquiry implies that anxiety does not, like rain, descend upon one capriciously but is explicable: it has causes that can be discovered (and therefore prevented and controlled).

Sometimes, if I have a strong hunch that there may be a delayed reaction to events of the hour, I suggest, toward the end of the session, a thought experiment involving projection into the future:

"We still have several minutes to go but I wonder if you might sit back, close your eyes, and imagine the hour is over and you are on your way home. What will you be thinking or feeling? How will you regard our session today? What feelings will you have about me or about the way we are relating?"

CHAPTER 67

Doctor, Take Away My Anxiety

If a patient is weighted down with anxiety and asks or pleads for relief, I generally find it useful to ask, "Tell me, what would be the perfect thing for me to say? What exactly could I say that would lead to your feeling better." I am, of course, not speaking to the patient's rational mind, but instead addressing the child part of the patient and asking for uncensored free associations.

In response to such a query, one patient told me, "I want you to tell me I'm the most beautiful, perfect baby in the world." I then told her exactly what she requested and together we examined the soothing effects of my words as well as other emerging feelings: her embarrassment for her childlike wishes and her great irritation that she had to tell me what to say. This exercise in self-soothing creates a certain paradox: the patient is thrown into a young, dependent state of mind by asking the therapist to utter magical words of relief but, at the same time, is forced to assume a position of autonomy by inventing the very words that will soothe her.

CHAPTER 68

On Being Love's Executioner

I do not like to work with patients who are in love. Perhaps it is because of envy—I too crave enchantment.
Perhaps it is because love and psychotherapy are funda-
mentally incompatible. The good therapist fights darkness and seeks illumination, while romantic love is
sustained by mystery and crumbles upon inspection. I
hate to be love's executioner.

A paradox: though these opening lines of *Love's Executioner* express my discomfort working with patients in
love, they have, nonetheless, prompted many patients
in love to consult me.

Of course, love comes in many forms and these lines refer
only to one particular type of love experience: the infatuated,
obsessed, highly magicalized state of mind that entirely pos-
sesses the individual.

Ordinarily such an experience is glorious, but there are
times when the infatuation causes more distress than pleasure.

Sometimes fulfillment of the love is forever elusive—for example, when one or both parties are married and unwilling to leave their marriage. Sometimes the love is not reciprocated—one person loves and the other shuns contact or wishes only a sexual relationship. Sometimes the loved one is entirely unobtainable—a teacher, a former therapist, the spouse of a friend. Often one may become so absorbed in love that he/she devotes much time waiting for some brief sight of the beloved to the neglect of all else—work, friends, family. A lover in an extramarital affair may withdraw from his/her spouse, may avoid intimacy in order to conceal the secret, may refuse couples therapy, may deliberately keep the marital relationship unsatisfying in order to diminish guilt and justify the affair.

However varied the circumstances, the experience is the same—the lover idealizes the beloved, is obsessed with her, often wishing nothing more than to spend the rest of his life basking in her presence.

To develop an empathic relationship with patients in love, you must not lose sight of the fact that their experience is quite wonderful: the ecstatic, blissful merger; the dissolving of the lonely "I" into the enchanted "we" may be one of the great experiences of the patient's life. It is generally advisable to express your appreciation of their state of mind and to refrain from criticism of the golden feeling surrounding the beloved.

No one ever put this dilemma better than Nietzsche, who, shortly after he "came to" from a passionate (but chaste) love affair with Lou Salome, wrote:

> One day a sparrow flew past me; and . . . I thought I'd seen an eagle. Now all the world is busy proving to me how wrong I am—and there's a proper European gossip about it. Well, who is better off? I, "the deluded one," as they say, who on account of this bird call dwelt for a

whole summer in a higher world of hope—or those, whom there is no deceiving?

So one must be delicate with a feeling that permits one to live in a "higher world of hope." Appreciate the patient's rapture but also help him prepare for its end. And it always ends. There is one true property of romantic love: it never stays—evanescence is a part of the nature of an infatuated love state. But be careful trying to rush its demise. Don't try to joust with love any more than you would with powerful religious beliefs—those are duels you cannot win (and there are similarities between being in love and experiencing religious ecstasy: One patient referred to his "Sistine Chapel state," another described his love as his celestial, imperishable condition). Be patient—leave it for the client to discover and express feelings about the irrationality of his feelings or disillusionment in the beloved. When any such expressions do occur, I remember the patient's words carefully. If and when he reenters that state again and re-idealizes the beloved, I may remind him of his comments.

At the same time I explore the experience much as I would any powerful emotional state. I say such things as "How wonderful for you . . . it's like coming to life again, isn't it? It's easy to understand why you don't want to give this up. Let's look at what permitted you to experience this now? . . . Tell me about your life in the weeks before this came upon you. When did you last feel love like this? What happened to that love?"

There is profit in focusing on the state of being in love rather than the person who is loved. It is the experience, the emotional state of loving—not the other person—that is so compelling. Nietzsche's phrase "One loves one's desire, not the desired" has often proved invaluable to me in my work with love-tormented patients.

Since most individuals know (though they try not to know)

that the experience will not persist forever, I try gently to introduce some long-range perspective and discourage the patient
from making any irreversible decision on the basis of feelings
that are likely to be evanescent.

Establish the goals of therapy early in your meetings. What
type of help is sought? Obviously there is something dysfunctional about the patient's experience or he wouldn't be consulting you. Is the patient asking for help in removing he himself
from the relationship? I often invoke the image of scales and
inquire about the balance of pleasure and displeasure (or hap-
piness and unhappiness) provided by the relationship. Sometimes a tally sheet helps illustrate the balance, and I ask
patients to keep a log, with several observation points a day, of
the number of times they think about the beloved, or even the
number of minutes or hours a day given to that pursuit.
Patients are sometimes astounded by the tallies, by how much
of their life is consumed by circular, repetitive thoughts and,
conversely, how little they participate in real-time life.

Sometimes I try to offer the patient perspective by discussing the nature and different forms of love. Erich Fromm's
timeless monograph, *The Art of Loving,* is a valuable resource
for patient and therapist alike. I often think of mature love as a
love of the being and the growth of the other, and most clients
will be sympathetic to this view. What, then, is the particular
nature of their love? Are they infatuated with someone whom,
at bottom, they do not really respect or someone who treats
them badly? Unfortunately, of course, there are those whose
love is intensified by not being treated well.

If they wish you to help them to get out of the relationship,
you might well remind them (and yourself) that release is arduous and slow. Occasionally an individual almost instantaneously emerges from an infatuation, much as the characters of
A Midsummer Night's Dream emerge from their enchantment,

but for the most part, individuals are tormented by yearnings for the beloved for many months. Sometimes years, even decades, pass before they can meet or even think of the other without twinges of desire or anxiety.

Nor is the dissolution a steady process. Setbacks occur—and nothing is more likely to bring about a setback than another encounter with the beloved. Patients offer many rationalizations for such new contact: they insist that they are over it now and that a cordial talk, a coffee, or lunch with the former beloved will help to clarify things, help them to understand what went wrong, help them establish a lasting adult friendship, or even permit them to say good-bye like a mature person. *None of these things is likely to come to pass.* Generally the individual's recovery is set back, much as a slip sets back a recovering alcoholic.

Don't get frustrated at setbacks—some infatuations are destined to go on for years. It's not a matter of weak will; there is something in the experience that touches the patient at very deep levels. Try to understand the crucial role played by the obsession in the individual's internal life. I believe that the love obsession often serves as a distraction, keeping the individual's gaze from more painful thoughts. Sooner or later I hope to arrive at the question: What would you be thinking about if you were not obsessed with . . . ?

CHAPTER 69

Taking a History

Early in their training, psychotherapy students are taught some systematic history-taking schemes. These schemes always include such items as the patient's presenting complaint, present illness, and history (including family, education, physical health, previous therapy, friendships, etc.). There are obvious advantages to a step-by-step method of collecting data. Physicians, for example, are trained to avoid oversight by taking a history and doing a physical examination in a highly routinized manner that consists of a systematic organ system review (nervous system, gastrointestinal system, genital-urinary system, cardiovascular system, musculoskeletal system).

Certain situations in therapy practice demand such a systematic method of collecting history—for example, in the first couple of sessions, when one is trying to get a quick read of the patient's life context; a time-limited consultation; or times when one must collect data quickly in order to make a succinct presentation to colleagues. However, once therapists gain experience, they rarely follow a systematic checklist of questions in the great bulk of their work in psychotherapy. Collecting data becomes intuitive and automatic. It does not precede therapy but is a part of the therapy itself. As Erik Erikson put it, "History taking is history making."

CHAPTER 70

A History of the Patient's Daily Schedule

Despite my reliance on an intuitive mode of collecting data, there is one particularly productive inquiry I always make in the first or second session: "Please give me a detailed account of your typical day."

I make sure everything is discussed, including eating and sleeping habits, dreaming, recreation, periods of discomfort and of joy, precise tasks at work, the use of alcohol and drugs, even reading, film, and TV preferences. If this inquiry is sufficiently detailed, therapists can learn a great deal, uncovering information that is often missed in other history-taking systems.

I listen to many things: eating habits, aesthetic preferences, leisure-time activities. In particular, I attend to how my patients' lives are peopled. With whom do they have regular contact? What faces do they regularly see? With whom do they have phone conversations or speak personally during the week? With whom do they have meals?

For example, in recent initial interviews this inquiry allowed me to learn of activities I might not otherwise have known for months: two hours a day of computer solitaire; three hours a night in Internet sex chat rooms under a different identity; massive procrastination at work and ensuing shame; a daily schedule so demanding that I was exhausted listening to it; a middle-aged woman's extended daily (sometimes hourly) phone calls with her father; a gay woman's long daily phone conversations with an ex-lover whom she disliked but from whom she felt unable to separate.

An inquiry into the minute details of the patient's life not only leads to rich material otherwise often missed but also gives a jump start to the bonding process. Such intense discussion of minute quotidian activities rapidly increases the sense of therapist-patient intimacy so necessary in the process of change.

CHAPTER 71

How Is the Patient's Life Peopled?

In a valuable study of interpersonal relationships, the psychologist Ruthellen Josselson uses a paper and pencil "solar system" instrument, instructing her subjects to represent themselves as a dot in the center of a page and the people in their life as objects circling them at various distances. The closer the dot to the center, the more central the relationship. Her particular study followed the positional changes in the circling satellites over a period of several years. While this instrument may be too cumbersome for everyday clinical use, it nonetheless serves as an excellent model for visualizing interpersonal patterns.

One of my major tasks in my early contacts is to find out how the patient's life is peopled. Much of that information may be obtained during a check of the patient's daily schedule, but I make certain to do a detailed inquiry into all the people who are important in the patient's life as well as any interpersonal contacts in a recent representative day. I also find it instructive to inquire about all the best friends, past and present, in the patient's life.

CHAPTER 72

Interview the Significant Other

N ever have I regretted interviewing some significant figure in the life of my patients—generally a spouse or
partner. In fact, at the end of such an interview I
invariably wonder, "Why did I wait so long?" or "Why don't I do
this more often?" When I hear patients describe their significant others, I create some mental image of the other person,
often forgetting that my information is highly skewed because
it has been filtered through the patient's imperfect and biased
eyes. But once I meet the significant others, they are fleshed in,
and I enter more fully into the life of my patient. Because I
meet the patient's partner in such an unusual situation, I'm
aware that I do not really "see" him/her, but that's not the
point—the point is that my image of the face and person of the
other permits me a richer encounter with my patient. Moreover, the partner may provide a new perspective and invaluable
information about the patient.

The significant others are, of course, threatened by an invitation to meet their partner's therapist. The partner appreciates

that the therapist who will be sizing them up has, understandably, a primary loyalty to the patient. But there is a strategy that rarely fails to diminish the threat and generally is effective in persuading the partner to come to the session. Instruct your patient in the following manner:

"John, please tell X that she could help me be more helpful to you. I'd like to obtain some of her feedback about you—especially some of the ways she might like to see you change. This is not an examination of her but a discussion of her observations of you."

Moreover, I recommend that the session be conducted in just that manner. Since I prefer to have no secret, outside knowledge of my patients, I always interview the significant other in the presence of my patient. Elicit the partner's feedback and suggestions for ideas of the changes the patient might make rather than conduct a personal interview of the partner. You will get a sufficiently complex picture of the partner just from the way he/she gives you feedback.

And I advise also that you don't turn the session into a couples session. When your primary loyalty is to one member of a pair with whom you have a therapy commitment, you are not the one to treat the couple. If you attempt couples therapy with a cargo of confidential information obtained from one member of the pair, you will soon be involved in withholding and duplicitous behavior. Couples therapy is best done by another therapist whose allegiance is to both participants equally.

CHAPTER 73

Explore Previous Therapy

If my patients have had previous therapy, I make a detailed inquiry into their experience. If the therapy was unsatisfactory, patients almost always cite their previous therapist's lack of engagement. The therapist, they say, was too distant, too uninvolved, too unsupportive, too impersonal. I have yet to hear a patient complain of a therapist being too revealing, too supportive, or too personal (with the exception, of course, of instances in which the patient and therapist have been sexually involved).

Once you become aware of the previous therapist's errors, then you can attempt to avoid repeating them. Make this explicit by checking in from time to time with simple direct inquiries. For example, "Mike, we've met for four sessions now and perhaps we should check into how you and I are doing. You've spoken of your feelings about Dr. X, your previous therapist. I wonder how that's playing out with me. Can you think of times you've had similar feelings about me or that you and I seemed to be moving into similar and unproductive patterns?"

If a patient has had a successful course of therapy in the past (and, for any number of reasons, is unable to continue with the same therapist), I believe it is equally important to explore what went right in therapy in order to incorporate those aspects in your current therapy. Don't expect these accounts of either successful or unsuccessful therapy to remain static: they generally change just as patients' views of other past events change. In time, patients may begin to recall positive effects of therapists they had at first vilified.

CHAPTER 74

Sharing the Shade of the Shadow

What do I remember of the seven hundred hours I spent on the couch in my first analysis? My brightest memory of my analyst, Olive Smith, that silent, patient listener, is of one day when I had placed myself on trial for greedily anticipating the money I might inherit when my parents died. I was doing a particularly good job at criticizing myself when, most uncharacteristically, she leapt into action and laid low the prosecution with one phrase: "That's just the way we're built."

It wasn't only that she reached out to comfort me, though I welcomed that. Nor that she normalized my base impulses. No, it was something else: It was the word *we*. It was the inference that she and I were alike, that she, too, had her shadow side.

I treasured her gift. And I have passed it on many times. I attempt to normalize my patients' darker impulses in any way I can. I reassure, I imitate Olive Smith in using *we*, I point out the ubiquity of certain feelings or impulses, I refer patients to appropriate reading material (for example, for sexual feelings I suggest the Kinsey, Masters and Johnson, or Hite reports).

Endeavor to normalize the shady side in any way possible. We therapists should be open to all our own dark, ignoble parts, and there are times when sharing them will enable patients to stop flagellating themselves for their own real or imaginary transgressions.

Once, after I had complimented a patient on the type of mothering she was providing for her two children, she grew visibly uncomfortable and announced gravely that she was going to tell me something she had never before shared, namely that after giving birth to her first child she had a strong inclination to walk out of the hospital and abandon her newborn. Though she wanted to be a mother she could not bear the idea of giving up so many years of freedom. "Show me the mother who hasn't had such feelings," I said. "Or the father. Though I love my children," I told her, "there were countless times that I deeply resented their encroachment upon my other tasks and interests in life."

The eminent British analyst D. W. Winnicott was particularly courageous in sharing his darker impulses, and a colleague of mine, when treating patients concerned about anger toward their children, often cites a Winnicott article in which are listed eighteen reasons why mothers hate their babies. Winnicott also cites the hostile lullabies mothers sing to babies, who fortunately do not understand the words. For example:

Rockabye, Baby, on the treetop,
When the wind blows the cradle will rock,
When the bough breaks the cradle will fall,
And down will come baby, cradle and all.

CHAPTER 75

Freud Was Not Always Wrong

Freud bashing has become fashionable. No contemporary reader can escape the recent scathing criticism condemning psychoanalytic theory as being as passé as the bygone culture from which it sprang. Psychoanalysis is attacked as a pseudoscience based on an outmoded scientific paradigm and eclipsed by recent advances in the neurobiology of dreaming and the genetics of schizophrenia and affective disorders. Furthermore, critics assert that it is a male-dominated fantasy of human development, teeming with sexism, and is constructed from distorted case histories and inaccurate, sometimes imaginary, observations.

So pervasive and pernicious has been this criticism that it has seeped even into therapy training programs, and a whole generation of mental health practitioners has been educated with a critical and wholly uninformed view of the man whose ideas comprise the very foundation of psychotherapy.

Let me suggest a thought experiment. Imagine you are in despair because of a failed relationship. You are besieged with hateful, disparaging thoughts about a woman whom, for months, you had idealized. You cannot stop thinking about her, you feel deeply, perhaps mortally, wounded, and you contemplate suicide—not only to end your pain but to punish the woman who caused it. You remain fixed in despair despite your friends' best efforts to console you. What would be your next step?

Most likely you would consider consulting a psychotherapist. Your symptoms—depression, anger, obsessive thoughts—all suggest not only that you are in need of therapy but that you would benefit considerably from it.

Now try a variation on that experiment. Imagine you have the same symptoms. But it is more than one hundred years ago, say 1882, and you live in Central Europe. What would you do? This is precisely the challenge I faced a few years ago while writing my novel *When Nietzsche Wept*. My plot called for Nietzsche to see a therapist in 1882 (the year in which he was in deep despair over the ending of his relationship with Lou Salome).

But who would be Nietzsche's therapist? After much historical research, it was apparent that there was no such creature in 1882—only 120 years ago. If Nietzsche had turned for help to a physician he would have been informed that lovesickness was not a medical problem and been advised to sojourn at Marienbad or one of the other baths of Europe for a water-and-rest cure. Or perhaps he might have been referred to a sympathetic clergyman for religious counseling. Practicing secular therapists? There were none! Though Liebault and Bernheim had a school of hypnotherapy in Nancy, France, they offered no psychotherapy per se, only hypnotic symptom removal. The field of secular psychotherapy had yet to be invented; it was awaiting the arrival of Freud, who in 1882 was still a medical intern and had not yet entered the field of psychiatry.

Not only did Freud single-handedly invent the field of psychotherapy but he did it in one fell swoop. In 1895 (in *Studies in Hysteria,* co-authored with Josef Breuer) he wrote an amazingly prescient chapter on psychotherapy that prefigures many of the major developments that were to occur over the next one hundred years. There Freud posits the fundamentals of our field: the value of insight and deep self-exploration and expression; the existence of resistance, transference, repressed trauma; the use of dreams and fantasies, role playing, free association; the need to address characterological problems as well as symptoms; and the absolute necessity of a trusting therapeutic relationship.

So instrumental to the education of the therapist do I consider these matters that for decades I offered at Stanford a Freud appreciation course in which I stressed two points: a reading of Freud's texts (rather than secondary sources) and an appreciation of his historical context.

Often popularizers are useful for students reading the works of thinkers who are unable to write clearly (or choose obfuscation)—for example, philosophers such as Hegel, Fichte, or even Kant or, in the field of psychotherapy, Sullivan, Fenichel, or Fairbairn. Not so with Freud. Though he did not win a Nobel Prize for scientific contribution, he was awarded the Goethe Prize for literary achievement. Throughout Freud's texts, his prose sparkles, even through the veil of translation. Indeed many of the clinical tales resemble those of a master storyteller.

In my teaching, I concentrate particularly on the first texts, *Studies in Hysteria,* selected sections of *The Interpretation of Dreams,* and *Three Essays on the Theory of Sexuality,* and sketch out his historical context—that is, the psychological zeitgeist of the late nineteenth century—which permits the student to realize how truly revolutionary were his insights.

One further point: We should not evaluate Freud's contributions on the basis of the positions advanced by the various

Freudian psychoanalytic institutes. Freud had many followers thirsty for some ritualized orthodoxy, and many analytic institutes adopted a conservative and static view of his work utterly out of keeping with his ever-changing creative and innovative disposition.

In my own professional development I have been exceedingly ambivalent toward traditional psychoanalytic training institutes. It seemed to me that the conservative analytic position of my day overvalued the importance of insight, particularly about psychosexual developmental issues, and furthermore was clueless about the importance of the human encounter in the therapeutic process. (Theodor Reik wrote: "The devil himself could not frighten many analysts more than the use of the word 'I.'") Consequently, I chose not to enter an analytic institute and, as I look back over my career, consider that one of the best decisions of my life. Although I encountered a great sense of professional isolation and uncertainty, I had the freedom to pursue my own interests and to think without restricting preconceptions.

My feelings today about the psychoanalytic tradition have changed considerably. Though I don't like many of the psychoanalytic institutional trappings and ideological positions, still those institutions are often the only game in town, the only place where serious technical psychodynamic issues are discussed by the best and brightest clinical minds in our field. Furthermore there has been, in my view, a recent salutary development in analytic thought and practice: that is, a rapidly growing analytic interest and literature on intersubjectivity and two-person psychology that reflects a new awareness of the crucial role of the basic human encounter in the process of change. To a significant degree, progressive analysts strive for greater genuineness and disclosure in their relationship with patients.

As managed care encourages shorter training (and, hence, cost cutting through cheaper therapist remuneration), therapists are more than ever in need of supplementary graduate clinical training. Psychoanalytic institutes (broadly defined—Freudian, Jungian, interpersonal, existential) offer, by far, the most thoughtful and thorough postgraduate dynamic therapy training. Furthermore, the institute culture offsets the isolation so inherent in therapeutic practice by providing a community of like minds, a group of colleagues facing similar intellectual and professional challenges.

Perhaps I am unduly alarmist but it seems to me that, in these days of relentless attack on the field of psychotherapy, the analytic institutes may become the last bastion, the repository of collected psychotherapy wisdom, in much the same way the church for centuries was the repository of philosophical wisdom and the only realm where serious existential questions—life purpose, values, ethics, responsibility, freedom, death, community, connectedness—were discussed. There are similarities between psychoanalytic institutes and religious institutions of the past, and it is important that we do not repeat the tendencies of some religious institutions to suppress other forums of thoughtful discourse and to legislate what thinkers are allowed to think.

CHAPTER 76

CBT Is Not What It's
Cracked Up to Be . . .
Or, Don't Be Afraid of the EVT Bogeyman

The concept of the EVT (empirically validated therapy) has had enormous recent impact—so far, all negative—on the field of psychotherapy. Only therapies that have been empirically validated—in actuality, this means brief cognitive-behavioral therapy (CBT)—are authorized by many managed-care providers. Graduate psychology schools granting master's and doctoral degrees are reshaping their curricula to concentrate upon the teaching of the EVTs; licensing examinations make certain that psychologists are properly imbued with the knowledge of EVT superiority; and major federal psychotherapy research funding agencies smile with particular favor upon EVT research.

All these developments create dissonance for many expert senior clinicians who are exposed daily to managed-care administrators insisting upon use of EVTs. Senior clinicians see an apparent avalanche of scientific evidence "proving" that their own approach is less effective than that offered by junior (and inexpensive) therapists delivering manualized CBT in astoundingly brief periods of time. In their guts they know this is wrong, they suspect the presence of smoke and mirrors, but have no evidentially based reply, and generally they have pulled in their horns and tried to go about their work hoping for the nightmare to pass.

Recent meta-analytic publications are restoring some balance. (I draw heavily from the excellent review and analysis of Weston and Morrison.) First, I urge clinicians to keep in mind that *nonvalidated* therapies are not *invalidated* therapies. Research, if it is to be funded, must have a clean design comparable to research testing drug efficacy. Design demands include "clean" patients (that is, patients with a single disorder without symptoms of any other diagnostic groups—a type of patient uncommonly seen in clinical practice), a brief therapy intervention, and a replicable, preferably manualized (that is, capable of being reduced to a step-by-step written manual) treatment mode. Such a design heavily favors CBT and excludes most traditional therapies that rely on an intimate (unscripted) therapist-patient relationship forged in genuineness and focusing on the here-and-now as it spontaneously evolves.

Many false assumptions are made in EVT research: that long-term problems can yield to brief therapy; that patients have only one definable symptom, which they can accurately report at the onset of therapy; that the elements of efficacious therapy are dissociable from one another; and that a written systematic procedural manual can permit minimally trained individuals to deliver psychotherapy effectively.

Analysis of results of EVT (Weston and Morrison) indicates far less impressive outcomes than has generally been thought. There is little follow-up at the end of one year and almost none at two years. The early positive response of EVTs (which is found in any therapeutic intervention) has led to a distorted picture of efficacy. The gains are not maintained and the percentage of patients who remain improved is surprisingly low. There is no evidence that therapist adherence to manuals positively correlates to improvement—in fact, there is evidence to the contrary. In general the implications of the EVT research have been extended far beyond the scientific evidence.

Naturalistic research on EVT clinical practice reveals that brief therapy is not so brief: clinicians using brief EVTs see patients for far more hours than is cited in reported research. Research indicates (to no one's surprise) that acute distress may be alleviated quickly but chronic distress requires far longer therapy, and characterological change the longest therapy course of all.

I can't resist raising one more mischievous point. I have a strong hunch (substantiated only anecdotally) that EVT practitioners requiring personal psychotherapeutic help do not seek brief cognitive-behavior therapy but instead turn to highly trained, experienced, dynamic, manual-less therapists.

CHAPTER 77

Dreams—
Use Them, Use Them, Use Them

Why do so many young therapists avoid working with dreams? My supervisees give me various answers. Many are intimidated by the nature of the dream literature—so voluminous, complex, arcane, speculative, and controversial. Students are often befuddled by dream symbol books and by the effluvia of vitriolic debates between Freudians, Jungians, gestaltists, and visionaries. Then, too, there is the rapidly developing literature on the new biology of dreams, which sometimes is sympathetic to dream work and sometimes dismissive by pronouncing dreams purely random and meaningless creations.

Others are frustrated and discouraged by the very form of dreams—by their ephemeral, cryptic, extravagant, and heavily disguised nature. Others, working in a managed-care-mandated brief-therapy framework, lack the time for dream work. Last, and perhaps most important, many young therapists have not had the experience of a probing personal therapy that itself profited from dream work.

I consider this inattention to dreams a great pity and a great loss for tomorrow's patients. Dreams can be an invaluable aid in effective therapy. They represent an incisive restating of the patient's deeper problems, only in a different language—a language of visual imagery. Highly experienced therapists have always relied on dreams. Freud considered them "the royal road to the unconscious." Although I agree, that is not, as I shall discuss, the main reason I find dreams so useful.

CHAPTER 78

Full Interpretation of a Dream?
Forget It!

Of all the misconceptions young therapists have about dream work, the most troublesome is the notion that one's goal should be to interpret a dream fully and accurately. That idea is without merit for the practice of psychotherapy, and I urge my students to abandon it.

Freud made one valiant and celebrated attempt at a full interpretation in his groundbreaking *Interpretation of Dreams* (1900), in which he thoroughly analyzed one of his dreams concerning a woman named Irma whom he had referred to a friend and colleague for surgery. Since the publication of the Irma dream, many theorists and clinicians have advanced new interpretations, and even now, one hundred years later, novel perspectives on that dream continue to appear in the psychoanalytic literature.

Even if it were possible to interpret a dream fully, it would not necessarily be a good use of the therapy hour. In my own practice I take a pragmatic approach to dreams and use them any way I can to facilitate therapy.

CHAPTER 79

Use Dreams Pragmatically:
Pillage and Loot

The fundamental principle underlying my work with dreams is to extract from them everything that expedites and accelerates therapy. Pillage and loot the dream, take out of it whatever seems valuable, and don't fret about the discarded shell. Consider this fearful dream that followed a patient's first session.

> "I was still in law school but I was trying a case in an open, large, crowded courtroom. I was still a woman but my hair was clipped short and I was dressed in a man's suit with high boots. My father, wearing a long white gown, was on trial and I was the prosecutor trying him on a rape charge. I knew at the time that I was being suicidal because he would ultimately track me down and kill me because of what I was doing to him."

The dream awakened her at three A.M. and was so frightening and so real that, terrified of a possible intruder, she raced around her home checking the locks on all windows and doors. Even as she related the dream to me a few hours later, she still felt apprehensive.

How do we loot this dream in the service of therapy? First, consider timing. Since we were just beginning therapy, my primary task was to forge a strong therapeutic alliance. Hence, my questions and comments focused primarily on those aspects of the dream that pertained to engagement and safety in the therapy situation. I asked such questions as "What do you make of putting your father on trial? I wonder, might that be related to telling me about him in our first therapy session? Do you feel it is dangerous to express yourself freely in this office? And your thoughts about the courtroom being open and crowded? I wonder, do you have concerns or doubts about the privacy and confidentiality of our meetings?"

Note that I did *not* attempt to interpret the dream. I did *not* inquire about many curious aspects of the dream: her gender confusion, her clothes, her father's white gown, his charge of rape. I tagged them, I stored them away. Perhaps I might turn back to these dream images in future sessions, but in the first stages of therapy I have another priority: I must attend to the frame of therapy—trust, safety, and confidentiality.

Another patient had this dream the night following our first session:

> "I went into a department store to get all my goods for a trip but there were things I was missing. They were down in the basement and I started to descend the stairs, which were dark and rickety. It was frightening. I saw a lizard. That was good: I like lizards—they're tough and haven't changed over the past hundred million years. Later I came upstairs and looked for my car, which was rainbow colored, but it was gone—maybe stolen. Then I

saw my wife in the parking lot, but my arms were too full
with packages and I was too rushed to go to her or to do
anything but gesture to her. My parents, too, were there
but they were pygmies and trying to build a campfire in
the parking lot."

The patient, a rigid and non-introspective forty-year-old
man, had long resisted therapy and agreed to consult me only
when his wife threatened to leave him unless he changed. His
dream was obviously influenced by the onset of therapy, which
is often depicted in dreams as a trip or journey. He feels unprepared for the therapy venture because the goods he needs are
in the basement (that is, his depths, his unconscious), but it is
difficult and eerie (the stairs are dark, frightening, and rickety).
Moreover, he is resistive to the therapy venture—he admires
lizards, which haven't changed for 100 million years. Or, perhaps, he is ambivalent about changing—his car is a risqué rainbow color but he cannot find it.

My task in the opening sessions? To help him engage in
therapy and to help him overcome his resistance to it. Hence, I
focused only on those components of the dream dealing with
the onset of therapy: the symbol of the journey, his sense of
unpreparedness and inadequacy, the dark, rickety stairs, the
descent, the lizard. I pointedly did not inquire about other
aspects of the dream: his wife and his difficulties in communi-
cating with her and his parents, who, changed into pygmies, lit
a fire in the parking lot. It's not that these aspects weren't
important—in later sessions we were to spend considerable
time exploring his relationships to his wife and parents—but in
the second session of therapy, there were other issues that took
precedence.

This dream, incidentally, illustrates an important aspect of
understanding the phenomenon, which Freud described in *The*

Interpretation of Dreams. Note that the dream deals with several abstract ideas—entering psychotherapy, fear of exploring the personal unconscious, feelings of inadequacy, uncertainty about whether or not to change. Yet dreams (aside from a very occasional auditory experience) are visual phenomena, and the agency of the mind that manufactures dreams must find a way to turn abstract ideas into visual form (a journey, rickety stairs descending into a basement, a lizard, a rainbow car).

ANOTHER CLINICAL EXAMPLE. A forty-five-year-old man, who had been in deep grief since his wife's death four years before, was a prolific dreamer and reported long, complex, and arresting dreams during each session. Triage was required: time did not permit investigation of all the dreams, and I had to select those that might facilitate our work on his chronic pathological grief. Consider these two dreams:

> "I was at my summer house and my wife was there, vague—a mere presence in the background. The house had a different kind of roof, a sod roof, and growing from it was a tall cypress—it was a beautiful tree but it was endangering the house and I had to cut it."

> "I was at home and fixing the roof of the house by placing some kind of ornament on it when I felt a big earthquake and could see the silhouette of the city shaking in the distance and saw two twin skyscrapers fall."

These dreams obviously related to his grief—his associations to "sod" as well as the roof "ornament" were his wife's grave and tombstone. It is not unusual for one's life to be depicted as a house in dreams. His wife's death and his unending grief were embodied by the cypress, which endangered his house and which therefore he had to cut. In the second dream his wife's death was represented by the earthquake, which collapsed the twin skyscrapers—the married couple. (This dream, incidentally, occurred years before the World Trade Center terrorist attack.) We had been working in therapy on the issues of coming to terms with the fact that the coupled state in which he had lived his life was no more, that his wife was truly dead, and that he had to let go, gradually detach from his wife, and reengage life. The reinforcement supplied by his dreams were instrumental in therapy—they represented to him a message from the fount of wisdom within him that it was time to fell the tree and to turn his attention to the living.

Sometimes a patient's dream contains an image so powerful, so overdetermined, containing so many layers of meaning, that it lodges in my mind and I refer to the dream again and again during the subsequent course of the therapy.

For example:

> "I was on the porch of my home looking through the window at my father sitting at his desk. I went inside and asked him for gas money for my car. He reached into his pocket, and as he handed me a lot of bills, he pointed to my purse. I opened my wallet and it already was crammed with money. Then I said that my gas tank was empty and he went outside to my car and pointed to the gas gauge, which said FULL."

The major theme in this dream was emptiness versus fullness. The patient wanted something from her father (and from me, since the room in the dream closely resembled the configuration of my office), but she couldn't figure out what she wanted. She asked for money and gasoline but her wallet was already stuffed with money and her gas tank was full. The dream depicted her pervasive sense of emptiness, as well as her belief that I had the power to fill her up if she could only discover the right question to ask. Hence she persisted in craving something from me—compliments, doting, special treatment, birthday presents—all the while knowing she was off the mark. My task in therapy was to redirect her attention—away from gaining supplies from another toward the richness of her own inner resources.

Another patient dreamed of herself as a hunchback and, studying her image in the mirror, tried to detach the tenacious hump, which ultimately changed into a screaming baby with long nails clutching and digging into her back. The idea of her inner, screaming, importunate baby greatly informed her future therapy.

Another patient, who felt trapped because she had to take care of an aged, demanding mother, dreamed that her own body had been transformed into the shape of a wheelchair.

A third patient, who entered therapy with amnesia about the events of the first ten years of his life and with remarkably little curiosity about his past, dreamed of walking along the Pacific coast and discovering a river that flowed backward, away from the ocean. He followed the river and soon came upon his dead father, a shabby homeless man standing before a cave entrance. A little farther along he discovered his grandfather in identical circumstances. This patient was haunted by death anxiety, and the dream image of the river running backward suggested an attempt to break the inexorable rush of time—to walk backward through time to discover his dead father and grandfather still living. He was much ashamed of the weaknesses and failures of his family, and the dream opened up an important seg-

ment of work on both his shame regarding his past and his terror of recapitulating it.

Another patient had a horrible nightmare:

> "My daughter and I were hiking and suddenly she
> began to sink. She had fallen into quicksand. I rushed to
> open my backpack to get my camera but had trouble
> unzipping the pack and then she was gone, sunk out of
> sight. It was too late. I couldn't save her."

A second dream that same night:

> "My family and I were trapped in a house by some
> older man who had killed people. We closed some heavy
> gates and then I went out to talk to the killer, who had a
> strangely familiar face and was dressed like some sort of
> royalty, and said: 'I don't want to offend you, but under
> the circumstances you have to appreciate our reluctance
> to let you in.'"

The patient was in a therapy group and shortly before the
dream had been confronted by several members who told him
he functioned as the group camera, an observer who did not
engage personally and did not bring his feelings into the group.
Incidentally, it is not unusual for a follow-up dream the same
night to express the same issue but in different image language.
(Freud referred to such dreams as companion dreams.) In our
therapy work we proceeded, as in all the other examples, to
focus on those parts of the dream that pertained to the current
stage of therapy—in this instance, the lack of engagement and
the restricted affect—and made no attempt to understand the
dream in its entirety.

CHAPTER 80

Master Some Dream
Navigational Skills

There are a number of well-tested aids to working with dreams. First, make it clear that you are interested in them. I make a point of inquiring about dreams in the first session (often in the context of exploring sleep patterns). I particularly inquire about repetitive dreams, nightmares, or other powerful dreams. Dreams occurring in the previous nights or last few nights usually yield more productive associations than older ones.

Toward the end of my first session, as I prepare the patient for therapy (see chapter 27) I include comments about the importance of dreams. If the patient claims not to dream or not to remember dreams, I give the standard instructions: "Keep a notepad by your bed. Jot down any part of the dream you remember in the morning or during the night. In the morning, review the dream in your mind, even before opening your eyes. Ignore the treacherous inner voice telling you not to bother writing it down because it is so vivid you won't forget it." With persistent nudging eventually (sometimes months later) even the most recalcitrant patients will begin to recall dreams.

Though I do not generally take notes during the session (aside from the initial meeting or two), I always write down descriptions of dreams—often they are complex and contain many small but pregnant details. Furthermore, important dreams may come up for discussion again and again during the course of therapy, and it is helpful to have a record of them. (Some therapists make a point of asking the patient to describe a dream a second time because the discrepancies between the two descriptions may provide leads about hot spots in the dream.) I find that asking the patient to repeat the dream in the present tense often brings it to life and plunges the patient back into the dream.

Usually my first question is about the dream affect. "What are the feelings you experience in the various parts of the dream? What is the emotional center of the dream?" Next I urge patients to select parts of the dream and associate freely to the content. Or I may select promising parts of the dream for them to mull upon. "Just take a couple of minutes," I instruct them, "and think about [some part of the dream] and let your mind wander freely. Think out loud. Say anything that comes into your mind. Don't censor, don't dismiss thoughts because they seem silly or irrelevant."

And, of course, I inquire about the relevant events of the day preceding the dream (the "day residue"). I have always found quite useful Freud's formulation that the dream borrows building blocks from the day residue, but that for images to be important enough to become incorporated into it, they must be reinforced by older, meaningful, affect-laden concerns.

Sometimes it is useful to consider all the figures in the dream to be aspects of the dreamer. The gestalt therapist Fritz Perls, who devised a number of powerful dream work techniqucs, considcrcd cvcrything in the dream to represent some aspect of the dreamer, and he would ask the dreamer to speak for each object in the dream. I remember watching him work effectively with a man who dreamed of his car being unable to start because of a bad spark plug. He asked the dreamer to play various parts—the car, the spark plug, the passengers—and to speak for each of them. The intervention threw light upon his procrastination and his crippling ambivalence; he did not want to go further with his life as he had defined it, and instead Perls helped him explore other paths not taken and another, unheeded, life calling.

CHAPTER 81

Learn About the Patient's
Life from Dreams

Another valuable use of dreams has little to do with the unconscious or the unraveling of dream distortion or discovering the meaning of the dream. The dream is an extraordinarily rich tapestry threaded through with poignant significant memories of the past. Simply culling those memories may often be a valuable endeavor. Consider this dream:

> "I am in a hospital room. The nurse wheels in a gurney covered with old newspapers and a baby with a bright crimson face. 'Whose baby?' I ask her. 'It's not wanted,' she answers. I pick it up and its diaper leaks all over me. I shout, 'I don't want it, I don't want it.'"

The patient's associations to the two emotion-laden points of this dream—the crimson baby and her shout of "I don't want it"—were rich and deeply informative. She mused about crimson babies and then thought of blue-and-yellow babies. The crimson baby made her think of an abortion she had had when she was a teenager and her parents' anger, rejection, and refusal to speak to her, other than to insist that she get an after-school job to stay out of further trouble. Then she thought of a girl she had known in the fourth grade who was a blue baby and had had heart surgery and had vanished, never to return to school. She had probably died, but since the patient's teachers never mentioned her again, she shuddered for years at the idea of death as a sudden arbitrary vanishing without a trace. "Blue" also meant depression, recalling her chronically depressed younger brothers. She had never wanted brothers and resented having had to share a room with them. And then she thought of "yellow baby" and her severe hepatitis when she was twelve and how abandoned by her friends she felt during her weeks of hospitalization. Yellow baby reminded her also of her son's birth and how terrified she was when he had been jaundiced at birth.

The other emotional part of the dream—her shouting "I don't want it"—had many implications for her: her husband not wanting her to have a baby, her feeling unwanted by her mother, her father sitting on her bed dozens of times and reassuring her excessively that she was a wanted child, her own rejection of her two younger brothers. She remembered how she, a ten-year-old white girl, had entered a recently integrated, mostly black school in the Bronx, where she was "unwanted" and attacked by the other students. Even though the school was dangerous, her father, a civil rights attorney, strongly supported school integration and refused to transfer her to a private school—another example, she thought, of how she and her best interests did not count to her parents. And, most relevant of all for our work, she felt she was unwanted by me; she considered her neediness so profound that she had to conceal it lest I get fed up and decide to bail out of treating her.

If not for her dream, many of these emotionally laden memories might never have surfaced in our therapy. The dream provided material for weeks of rich discussions.

The persons appearing in dreams often may be composite figures—they don't quite look like any one person but there are parts of many people in them. I often ask patients, if they still see the dream and the person in their mind's eye, to focus on the face and to free-associate. Or I may suggest they close their eyes and allow the face to transform into other faces and describe to me what they see. In this manner, I have often learned of all sorts of vanished individuals—uncles, aunts, best friends, ex-lovers, teachers—who played some important but forgotten role in the patient's life.

Sometimes it is useful to react spontaneously, to express some of your own loose associations to the dream. Of course, that may bias the work, since it is the patient's associations, not yours, that lead to a truer vision of the dream, but since I'm concerned with what advances the therapy work, not with some illusory genuine interpretation of the dream, that doesn't trouble me. Consider, for example, the following dream:

> "I'm in your office but it is much larger and our chairs seem large and very far apart. I try to get closer but instead of walking I roll across the floor to you. You then sit on the floor, too, and then we continue to talk, with you holding my feet. I tell you I don't like you smelling my feet. You then put my feet next to your cheek. I like that."

The patient could do very little with this dream. I inquired about my smelling her feet and she described her fears that I would see her darker, unpleasant side and reject her. But the rest of the dream appeared mysterious and opaque to her. Then I expressed my reaction: "Margaret, this seems like a very young dream—the large room and furniture, your rolling over to me, the two of us being on the floor, my smelling your feet, holding them against my cheek—the whole ambiance of the dream makes me feel it is from a very young child's point of view."

My comments struck some important chord, for on the way home after the session, she was flooded with forgotten memories of the way she and her mother had often massaged each other's feet while having long, intimate talks. She had had a highly troubled relationship with her mother and for many months of therapy she had held the position that her mother had been relentlessly distant and that they had shared few physically intimate moments. The dream told us otherwise and ushered in the next stage of therapy, in which she reformulated her past and recast her parents in softer, more human hues.

Another dream that announced or ushered in a new phase of therapy was recounted by a patient who was amnesic for much of his childhood and curiously uncurious about his past.

"My father was still alive. I was in his home and was looking in some old envelopes and notebooks that I wasn't supposed to be opening until he was dead. But then I noticed a green light blinking on and off, which I could see right though one of the sealed envelopes. It was like my cell phone blinking."

The awakening of the patient's curiosity and the call from his inner self (the blinking green light) instructing him to turn his gaze to his relationship with his father are easily evident in this dream.

A final example of a dream opening up new vistas for therapy:

"I was getting dressed for a wedding but couldn't find my dress. I was given a stack of wood to build the wedding altar but I had no idea how to do it. Then my mother was braiding my hair into cornrow braids. Then we were sitting on a sofa and her head was very close to my face and I could feel her whiskers and then she disappeared and I was alone."

The patient had no notable associations to this dream—especially to the odd image of the cornrow braid (with which she had no personal experience)—until the next evening, when, lying in her bed near sleep, she suddenly remembered that Martha, long forgotten, but her best friend during the first through third grades, had cornrow braids! She recounted an episode in the third grade when her teacher rewarded her good class work by granting her the privilege of putting up the class Halloween decorations and permitting her to select another student to assist her. Thinking it would be a good idea to broaden her friendships, she selected another girl rather than Martha.

"Martha never spoke to me again," she said sadly, "and that was the last best friend I ever had." She then proceeded to give me a history of her lifelong loneliness and all the potential intimacies that she somehow sabotaged. Another association (to the dream image of the head close to her) was of her fourth-grade teacher putting her head very close to her, as though she were going to murmur something tender, but instead hissing, "Why did you do it?" The whiskers in the dream brought to mind my beard and her fear of allowing me to get too close to her. The patient's reconnecting with the dream as she approached sleep the following night is an example of state-associated memories—a not uncommon phenomenon.

CHAPTER 82

Pay Attention to the First Dream

Ever since Freud's 1911 paper on the first dream in psychoanalysis, therapists have had particular respect for the patient's first dream in therapy. This initial dream, Freud believed, is often a priceless document, which offers an exceptionally revealing view of core problems because the dream-weaver within the patient's unconscious is still naïve and has its guard down. (For rhetorical reasons only, Freud sometimes spoke of the agency of the mind that elaborates dreams as though it were an independent homunculus.) Later in therapy, when the therapist's dream-interpretive abilities become evident, our dreams become more complex and obfuscating.

Remember the prescience of the two first dreams in chapter 79. In the first a woman attorney prosecuted her father for rape. In the second a man going on a long journey shopped for provisions in a department store in which he had to descend a dark stairway. Here are some others.

A patient whose husband was dying of a brain tumor had this dream the night before her first therapy session:

"I'm still a surgeon, but I'm also a grad student in English. My preparation for a course involves two different texts, an ancient and a modern one, each with the same name. I am unprepared for the seminar because I haven't read either text. I especially haven't read the old, first text, which would have prepared me for the second."

When I asked whether she knew the name of the texts, she answered, "Oh yes, I remember it clearly. Each book, the old and the new, was entitled *The Death of Innocence*."

This extremely prescient dream adumbrated much of our future work. The ancient and the modern texts? She was certain she knew what they represented. The ancient text was her brother's death in a traffic accident twenty years earlier. Her husband's death to come was the modern text. The dream told us that she was not going to be able to deal with her husband's death until she had come to terms with the loss of her brother, a loss that had marked her for life, that had exploded all her young innocent myths about divine providence, the safety of home, the presence of justice in the universe, the sense of order dictating that the old die before the young.

First dreams often express patients' expectations or fears about the impending therapy. My own first dream in analysis is still fresh in my mind after forty years:

"I am lying on a doctor's examining table. The sheet is too small to cover me properly. I can see a nurse inserting a needle into my leg—my shin. Suddenly there's an explosive hissing, gurgling sound—*WHOOOOOSH*."

The meaning of the center of the dream—the loud *whoosh*—was instantly clear to me. As a child I was plagued with chronic sinusitis, and every winter my mother took me to

Dr. Davis for a sinus draining and flushing. I hated his yellow teeth and the one fishy eye peering at me though the center of the circular mirror attached to the headband that otolaryngologists used to wear. I remembered those visits: his inserting a cannula into my sinus foramen, my feeling a sharp pain, then hearing a deafening *whooooosh* as the injected saline flushed out my sinus. I remembered my observing the quivering, disgusting contents of the chrome semicircular drainage pan and thinking that some of my brains had been washed out along with the pus and mucus.

All my fears of my upcoming analysis were expressed in the dream: that I would be exposed (the too-small sheet) and be painfully penetrated (the needle insertion), that I would lose my mind, be brainwashed, and suffer a grievous injury to a long, firm body part (depicted as a shinbone).

A female patient once dreamed the night before her first session that I would break all the windows in her home and give her an anesthetic injection in the heart. Our discussion of the anesthetic injection in the heart disclosed that, though she was a highly successful scientist, she was strongly tempted to overturn her career and try to become a painter. She was afraid that my therapy would put her artist heart to sleep and force her to continue her more rational but deadened life trajectory.

These dreams remind us that misconceptions about therapy are deep and tenacious. Don't be misled by appearances. Assume that new patients have fears and confusion about therapy and make certain to prepare each patient for the course of psychotherapy.

CHAPTER 83

Attend Carefully to Dreams About the Therapist

Of all the dreams offered by patients, I believe there are none more valuable to the therapy enterprise than dreams involving the therapist (or some symbolic stand-in for the therapist). These dreams represent great potential for therapeutic payoff and, as the following examples show, merit careful harvesting.

A patient dreamed the following:

> "I am in your office and you say to me, 'You're an odd bird. I've never seen anything like you before.'"

As usual, I inquired about the feeling tone of the dream. "Warm and cozy," he responded. This patient, who had a number of unusual ritualistic obsessive-compulsive practices, characteristically undervalued his many assets—his intelligence, wide range of knowledge and interests, his dedication to a life of service. He persuaded himself that I would be interested only in his oddity. Much as I might take an interest in a freak in a circus sideshow. The dream led us into the important area of his lifelong practice of cultivating quirkiness as a mode of interacting with others. Soon the trail led to his self-contempt and his fears that he would be dismissed by others because of his emptiness, shallowness, and sadistic fantasies.

A dream from another patient:

> "You and I are having sex in my sixth-grade classroom. I am undressed but you still have all your clothes on. I ask whether it was satisfying enough for you."

This patient had been sexually abused by a teacher in grammar school and had been exceedingly upset by discussing it in our recent sessions. Our work on the dream opened up a number of trenchant issues. She had felt sexually stimulated by our intimate discussion about sex. "Talking about sex with you is something like having sex with you," she said, and suspected that I, too, had been stimulated and had been obtaining voyeuristic pleasure from her disclosures. She discussed her discomfort with the inequality of disclosure—in our sessions she undressed while I remained hidden. The question raised in the dream of whether I was being sexually satisfied reflected her fear that the only thing she had to give was sex and that I would abandon her if she failed to provide it for me.

Another dream:

> "I was in a split-level house. There was a ten-year-old girl trying to break it apart, and I fight her off. Then I see a yellow Goodwill truck driving up and crashing again and again against the foundations of my room. I hear the words, 'The helping hand strikes again.'"

My role in this dream as the Goodwill truck threatening the foundations of her house is unmistakable. But just in case we miss it, the dream redundantly adds, "The helping hand strikes again." The patient, a repressed, constricted woman, came from an alcoholic family much invested in keeping secrets from the community. The dream expressed her fears of exposure as well as an admonition to me to be gentle and careful.

Another clinical example. Toward the end of the therapy a female patient dreamed the following:

> "We're attending a conference together at a hotel. At some point you suggest that I get a room adjoining yours so we can sleep together. So I go to the hotel registration desk and arrange for my room to be moved. Then a short time later you change your mind and tell me it is not a good idea, after all. So I go back to the desk to cancel the transfer. But it is too late: all of my things have been moved to the new room. But then it turns out that the new room is a much nicer room—larger, higher, better view. And, numerologically, the room number, 929, is a far more propitious number."

This dream appeared as the patient and I were beginning to discuss termination. It expressed her view that I was at first seductive (that is, the dream image of my suggesting she and I take adjoining rooms and sleep together) and that she responded by getting closer to me (she switched rooms) but then, when I changed my mind about having sex with her, she could not get her old room back—that is, she had already undergone some irreversible change. Furthermore, the change was for the best—the new room was a superior room with salubrious numerological implications. This patient was an exceptionally beautiful woman who exuded sexuality and had in the past related to all men via some form of explicit or sublimated sexuality. The dream suggests that sexual energy between us may have been essential for the therapeutic bond to be forged, which, once in place, facilitated irreversible changes.

Another clinical example:

> "I am in your office. I see a beautiful dark-eyed woman with a red rose in her hair reclining on a sofa. As I approach, I realize that the woman is not as she had seemed: her sofa is really a bier, her eyes are dark not with beauty but with death, and her crimson rose is no flower but a bloody mortal wound."

This patient (described extensively in *Momma and the Meaning of Life*) had often expressed her reluctance to engage me as a real person. In our discussion about the dream she said, "I know that I am this woman and anyone approaching me will, ipso facto, be introduced to death—another reason to keep you away, another reason for you not to get too close."

The dream led us into the theme of her being cursed: so many men she had loved had died that she believed she carried death with her. It was the reason she refused to let me materialize as a person—she wanted me outside of time, without a life narrative consisting of a trajectory with a beginning and, of course, most of all, an end.

My notebooks are crammed with numerous other examples of my appearance in my patients' dreams. One patient dreamed of urinating upon my watch, another of wandering through my home, meeting my wife, and becoming part of my family. As I age more, patients dream of my absence or death. In the introduction I cited a dream of a patient who upon entering my deserted office found only a hat rack holding my cobweb-filled Panama hat. Another came into my office to find a librarian seated at my desk who informed her that my office had been converted into a memorial library. Every therapist can supply other examples.

CHAPTER 84

Beware the Occupational Hazards

The cozy setting of psychotherapy practice—comfortable armchairs, tasteful furnishings, gentle words, the sharing, the warmth, the intimate engagement—often obscures the occupational hazards. Psychotherapy is a demanding vocation, and the successful therapist must be able to tolerate the isolation, anxiety, and frustration that are inevitable in the work.

What a paradox it is that psychotherapists, who so cherish their patients' pursuit of intimacy, should experience isolation as a major professional hazard. Yet therapists too often are solitary creatures, spending all their working day cloistered in one-to-one sessions and rarely seeing colleagues unless they make a strenuous effort to build collegial activities into their life. Yes, of course, the therapist's workaday one-to-one sessions are drenched in intimacy, but it is a form of intimacy insufficient to support the therapist's life, an intimacy that does not provide the nourishment and renewal that emanate from deep, loving relationships with friends and family. It is one thing to be for the other, but quite another thing to be in relationships that are equally for oneself and the other.

Too often, we therapists neglect our personal relationships. Our work becomes our life. At the end of our workday, having given so much of ourselves, we feel drained of desire for more relationship. Besides, patients are so grateful, so adoring, so idealizing, we therapists run the risk of becoming less appreciative of family members and friends, who fail to recognize our omniscience and excellence in all things.

The therapist's worldview is in itself isolating. Seasoned therapists view relationships differently, they sometimes lose patience with social ritual and bureaucracy, they cannot abide the fleeting shallow encounters and small talk of many social gatherings. While traveling, some therapists avoid contact with others or conceal their profession because they are put off by the public's distorted responses toward them. They are weary not only of being irrationally feared or devaluated but of being overvaluated and deemed capable of mind-reading or of rendering curbstone solutions to multifarious problems.

Although therapists should be inured to the idealization or devaluation they face in their everyday work, they rarely are. Instead, they often experience unsettling ripples of self-doubt or grandiosity. These shifts in self-confidence, indeed all changes in inner states, must be carefully scrutinized by therapists lest they interfere with the therapy work. Disruptive life experiences encountered by the therapist—relationship strains, birth of children, child-rearing stresses, bereavement, marital discord and divorce, unforeseen reversals, life calamities, illnesses—all may dramatically increase the strain and the difficulty of doing therapy.

All of these professional hazards are much influenced by one's work schedule. Therapists who are under personal financial pressures and schedule forty to fifty hours a week are far more at risk. I've always considered psychotherapy as more of a calling than a profession. If accumulating wealth, rather than being of service, is one's primary motivation, then the life of a psychotherapist is not a good career choice.

Therapist demoralization is related also to one's range of practice. Overspecialization, especially in clinical areas loaded with great pain and desolation—for example, working with the dying, or the severely chronically impaired or psychotic—puts the therapist much at risk; I believe that balance and diversity in one's practice vastly contribute to a sense of renewal.

Earlier, when I discussed the transgression of sexual involvement with patients, I pointed out the similarity of the therapist-patient relationship to any exploitable relationship containing a power differential. But there exists a major difference that inheres in the very intensity of the therapy endeavor. The therapeutic bond can become so strong—so much is revealed, so much asked, so much given, so much understood—that love arises, not only from the patient but also from the therapist, who must keep love in the realm of *caritas* and prevent its slippage into eros.

Of all the stresses in the life of the psychotherapist, there are two that are particularly catastrophic: the suicide of a patient and a malpractice lawsuit.

If we work with troubled patients, we will always have to live with the possibility of suicide. Approximately 50 percent of senior therapists have faced the suicide, or a serious suicide attempt, of a current or past patient. Even the most mature and seasoned therapist will be tormented by shock, sadness, guilt, feelings of incompetence, and anger at the patient.

Equally painful emotions are experienced by the therapist facing a malpractice lawsuit. In today's litigious world, competence and integrity are no protection to the therapist: almost every competent therapist I know has, at least once, been exposed to a lawsuit or the threat of lawsuit. Therapists feel deeply betrayed by the experience of litigation. After dedicating themselves to a life of service, always striving to enhance the growth of their patients, therapists are profoundly shaken and sometimes permanently changed by the experience. A new and unpleasant thought occurs to them when they do an initial evaluation: "Will this person sue me?" I personally know therapists who were so demoralized by a malpractice suit that they decided upon early retirement.

Sixty years ago, Freud advised therapists to return to personal analysis every five years because of frequent exposure to primitive repressed material, which he likened to dangerous exposure to X rays. Whether or not one shares his concern that the therapist's repressed instinctual demands might be stirred up, it is hard to disagree with his belief that the inner work of therapists must continue in perpetuity.

Personally I have found a psychotherapist support group to be a mighty bulwark against many of these hazards. For the past ten years I have attended a leaderless group that consists of eleven male therapists of approximately the same age and experience and meets for ninety minutes every other week. But none of these particular group properties is essential: for example, for many years I led a successful weekly therapy group for psychotherapists of mixed age and gender. What is essential is that the group offer a safe, trusting arena for the sharing of the stresses of personal and professional life. Nor does it matter what the group is called—that is, whether it is a "therapy group" or a "support group" (which happens to be therapeutic for its members).

If there is no confounding interpersonal incompatibility among the members, a group of experienced clinicians needs no professional leader. In fact, the absence of a designated leader may enable the membership to exercise their own sharply honed skills more fully. A group of less experienced therapists, on the other hand, may benefit from an experienced leader serving both as facilitator and mentor. Forming a support group is easier than one might think. All that is required is the resolve of one or two dedicated individuals who generate a list of compatible colleagues, contact them, and arrange for the time and place of a planning session.

In my view, groups are a powerful vehicle for generating support and personal change. Couple that with the skills and resources inherent in a gathering of experienced clinicians and it is obvious why I so passionately urge therapists to avail themselves of this opportunity.

CHAPTER 85

Cherish the Occupational Privileges

I rarely hear my therapist colleagues complain that their lives lack meaning. Life as a therapist is a life of service in which we daily transcend our personal wishes and turn our gaze toward the needs and growth of the other. We take pleasure not only in the growth of our patient but also in the ripple effect—the salutary influence our patients have upon those whom they touch in life.

There is extraordinary privilege here. And extraordinary satisfaction, too.

In the preceding discussion of professional hazards I described the arduous, never-ending self-scrutiny and inner work required by our profession. But that very requirement is more privilege than burden because it is an inbuilt safeguard against stagnation. The active therapist is always evolving, continuously growing in self-knowledge and awareness. How can one possibly guide others in an examination of the deep structures of mind and existence without simultaneously examining oneself? Nor is it possible to ask a patient to focus upon interpersonal relatedness without examining one's own modes of relating. I receive plenty of feedback from patients (that I am, for example, withholding, rejecting, judgmental, cold and aloof), which I must take seriously. I ask myself whether it fits my internal experience and whether others have given me similar feedback. If I conclude that the feedback is accurate and illuminates my blind spots, I feel grateful and thank my patients. Not to do so, or to deny the veracity of an accurate observation, is to undermine the patient's view of reality and to engage not in therapy but in anti-therapy.

We are cradlers of secrets. Every day patients grace us with their secrets, often never before shared. Receiving such secrets is a privilege given to very few. The secrets provide a backstage view of the human condition without social frills, role playing, bravado, or stage posturing. Sometimes the secrets scorch me and I go home and hold my wife and count my blessings. Other secrets pulsate within me and arouse my own fugitive, long-forgotten memories and impulses. Still others sadden me as I witness how an entire life can be needlessly consumed by shame and the inability to forgive oneself.

Those who are cradlers of secrets are granted a clarifying lens through which to view the world—a view with less distortion, denial, and illusion, a view of the way things really are. (Consider, in this regard, the titles of books written by Allen Wheelis, an eminent psychoanalyst: *The Way Things Are, The Scheme of Things, The Illusionless Man.*)

When I turn to others with the knowledge that we are all (therapist and patient alike) burdened with painful secrets— guilt for acts committed, shame for actions not taken, yearnings to be loved and cherished, deep vulnerabilities, insecurities, and fears—I draw closer to them. Being a cradler of secrets has, as the years have passed, made me gentler and more accepting. When I encounter individuals inflated with vanity or self-importance, or distracted by any of a myriad of consuming passions, I intuit the pain of their underlying secrets and feel not judgment but compassion and, above all, connectedness. When I was first exposed, at a Buddhist retreat, to the formal meditation of loving-kindness, I felt myself much at home. I believe that many therapists, more than is generally thought, are familiar with the realm of loving-kindness.

Not only does our work provide us the opportunity to transcend ourselves, to evolve and to grow, and to be blessed by a clarity of vision into the true and tragic knowledge of the human condition, but we are offered even more.

We are intellectually challenged. We become explorers immersed in the grandest and most complex of pursuits—the development and maintenance of the human mind. Hand in hand with patients, we savor the pleasure of great discoveries— the "aha" experience when disparate ideational fragments suddenly slide smoothly together into coherence. At other times we are midwife to the birth of something new, liberating, and elevating. We watch our patients let go of old self-defeating patterns, detach from ancient grievances, develop zest for living, learn to love us, and, through that act, turn lovingly to others. It is a joy to see others open the taps to their own founts of wisdom. Sometimes I feel like a guide escorting patients through the rooms of their own house. What a treat it is to watch them open doors to rooms never before entered, discover new wings of their house containing parts in exile—wise, beautiful, and creative pieces of identity. Sometimes the first step of that process is in dream work, when both the patient and I marvel at the emergence from darkness of ingenious constructions and luminous images. I imagine creative writing teachers must have similar experiences.

Last, it has always struck me as an extraordinary privilege to belong to the venerable and honorable guild of healers. We therapists are part of a tradition reaching back not only to our immediate psychotherapy ancestors, beginning with Freud and Jung and all *their* ancestors—Nietzsche, Schopenhauer, Kierkegaard—but also to Jesus, the Buddha, Plato, Socrates, Galen, Hippocrates, and all the other great religious leaders, philosophers, and physicians who have, since the beginning of time, ministered to human despair.

Notes

p. xiv—Erikson, Erik, *Identity: Youth and Crisis* (New York: W. W. Norton, 1968), pp. 138–39.

p. 1—Karen Horney, *Neurosis and Human Growth* (New York: W. W. Norton, 1950).

p. 5—C. P. Rosenbaum, personal communication, 2001.

p. 6—André Malraux, *Antimemoirs* (New York: Holt, Rinehart, and Winston, 1968), p. 1.

p. 6—Arthur Schopenhauer, parerga and paralipomena, Volume 2, translated by E. Payne (Clarendon Press. Oxford. 1974) p. 292

p. 6,7—Arthur Schopenhauer, The *Complete Essays of Schopenhauer,* trans T. Bailey Saunders (New York: Wiley, 1942),p.2

p. 7—ibid–p.298

p.8—Hermann Hesse, *The Glass Bead Game: Magister Ludi*, Richard Winston.

p. 15—Ram Dass, oral communication, 1988.

p. 18—Carl Rogers, "The Necessary and Sufficient Conditions of Psychotherapeutic Personality Change," *Journal of Consulting Psychology* 21 (1957): 95–103.

p. 21—Irvin Yalom, *Every Day Gets a Little Closer* (New York: Basic Books, 1974).

p. 21—Terence, *Lady of Andros, Self-Tormentor & Eunuch*, vol. 1, trans. John Sargeant (Cambridge: Harvard University Press, 1992).

p. 29—This dream is discussed in *Momma annd the Meaning of Life* (New York: Basic Books, 1999.)

p. 31—This incident discussed in *Momma and the Meaning of Life* (New York: Basic Books, 1999.)

p. 63—K. Benne, "History of the T-group in the laboratory setting," in *T-Group Theory and Laboratory Method*, ed. L. Bradford, J. Gibb, K. Benne (New York : John Wiley, 1964), pp. 80–135.

p. 64—Irvin Yalom, *Inpatient Group Psychotherapy* (New York: Basic Books, 1983).

p. 64—Irvin Yalom, *Every Day Gets a Little Closer* (New York: Basic Books, 1974).

p. 73—Irvin Yalom, *Love's Executioner* (New York: Basic Books, 1989).

p. 76—Sigmund Freud, *Studies in Hysteria* (New York: Basic books, 2001).

p. 79—Irvin Yalom, "Group Therapy and Alcoholism," *Annals of the New York Academy of Sciences* 233 (1974): 85–103.

p. 81—Yalom, S. Bloch, S. Brown, "The Written Summary as a Group Psychotherapy Technique," *Archives of General Psychiatry* 32 (1975): 605–13.

p. 81—Sándor Ferenczi, *The Clinical Diaries of Sándor Ferenczi*, ed. Judith Dupont (Cambridge: Harvard University Press, 1995).

p. 82—Irvin Yalom, *Lying on the Couch* (New York: Basic Books, 1996).

p. 89—Peter Lomas, *True and False Experience* (New York: Taplinger, 1993), pp. 15–16.

p. 104—Friedrich Nietzsche, *Thus Spake Zarathustra* (New York: Penguin Books, 1961), p. 85.

p. 106—Louis Fierman, ed., *Effective Psychotherapy: The Contributions of Helmut Kaiser* (New York: The Free Press, 1965), pp. 172–202.

p. 106—Irvin Yalom, *When Nietzsche Wept* (New York: Basic Books, 1972).

p. 108—Harry Stack Sullivan, *The Psychiatric Interview* (New York: Norton, 1988).

p. 112—J. Luft, *Group Processes: An Introduction to Group Dynamics* (Palo Alto, Calif.: National Press, 1966).

p. 128—I. Yalom, M. Liebermann, "Bereavement and Heightened Existential Awareness," *Psychiatry,* 1992.

p. 131—Irvin Yalom, *Existential Psychotherapy* (New York: Basic Books, 1980), p. 146.

p. 148—J. Gardner, *Grendel* (New York: Random House, 1989).

p. 149—Martin Heidegger, *Being and Time* (New York: Harper and Row, 1962), p. 294.

p. 175—Friedrich Nietzsche, *The Gay Science* (New York: Vintage Books, 1974).

p. 175—Friedrich Nietzsche, *The Will to Power* (New York: Vintage Books, 1967), p. 272.

p. 176—Friedrich Nietzsche, *The Will to Power* (New York: Vintage Books, 1967), p. 267.

p. 201—Irvin Yalom, *Love's Executioner* (New York: Basic Books, 1989), p. 15.

p. 202–3—Friedrich Nietzsche, Letter to P. Gast 4 August 1882, cited by P. Fuss and H. Shapiro, in *Nietzsche: A Self-portrait from His Letters* (Cambridge: Harvard University Press, 1971), p. 63.

p. 203—Friedrich Nietzsche, *Beyond Good and Evil* (New York: Vintage Books, 1989), p. 95.

p. 204—Erich Fromm, *The Art of Loving* (New York: Perennial Classics, 2000).

p. 207—Erik Erikson, personal communication, 1970.

p. 210—Ruthellen Josselson, *The Space Between Us* (New York: Sage, 1995), p. 201.

p. 216—D. W. Winnicott, "Hate in the Counter-transference," *International Journal of Psychoanalysis* 30 (1949): 69.

p. 219—Sigmund Freud, *Studies in Hysteria* (New York: Basic Books Classics, 2000).

p. 223—Drew Weston and Kate Morrison, "How Empirically Valid Are EVPs? A Critical Appraisal," *The Journal of Consulting and Clinical Psychology*, in press.

p. 243—Sigmund Freud, *The Handling of Dream Interpretations*, standard edition, vol. 12 (London: the Hogarth Press, 1958), p. 91.

p. 243—These two dreams are described in *Momma and the Meaning of Life* (New York: Basic Books, 1999).

p. 249—Irvin Yalom, *Momma and the Meaning of Life* (New York: Basic Books, 1999), pp. 83–154.

p. 254—Sigmund Freud, *Analysis Terminable and Interminable*, Standard Edition, vol. 23, p. 249